The
SELF-CARE
Project

The
SELF-CARE
Project

Jayne Hardy

First published in Great Britain in 2017 by Orion Spring
an imprint of The Orion Publishing Group Ltd
Carmelite House, 50 Victoria Embankment
London EC4Y 0DZ

An Hachette UK Company

10 9 8 7 6 5 4

Illustrations by Dominic Hardy

A CIP catalogue record for this book is
available from the British Library.

ISBN: 978 1 4091 7758 6

Printed in Italy

Every effort has been made to ensure that the information in the book
is accurate. The information in this book may not be applicable in
each individual case so it is advised that professional medical advice
is obtained for specific health matters and before changing any
medication or dosage. Neither the publisher nor author accepts any legal
responsibility for any personal injury or other damage or loss arising
from the use of the information in this book. In addition if you are
concerned about your diet or exercise regime and wish to change them,
you should consult a health practitioner first.

ORION
SPRING

www.orionbooks.co.uk

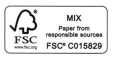

Contents

For you, and for me.
Dedicated to Domski, Pegs, Mother Hubbs, Clairie and Windog.

Introduction

Self-care is accessible and applicable to everyone, but it's one thing knowing the benefits and quite another to prioritise it.

Life can be noisy. It can be exhausting too. There are too many things vying for our attention, and sometimes we inadvertently forget how important our wellbeing is. It's so easily done because the external noise is so, so loud. It comes at us from many different angles, and it demands our attention.

And so, we give it our attention.

We place other people's needs and wants ahead of our own, and we get sidelined.

We live in a fast-paced world rife with social media images of perfection. We don't feel good enough or as though we're doing enough. We compare where we are with heavily filtered snapshots of a single moment in time and wonder where we're going so wrong.

Drowning out the noise and tuning into your wants and needs isn't easy.

We forget what it is that nourishes us. We forget that we matter. Our actions tell everyone else how important they are and where we come in the pecking order – usually near the bottom, a mere afterthought. So many of us have danced to other people's tunes throughout our lives. We live to their ideals and expectations, allow them to shape and design our lives. Our boundaries become wonky. We lose a sense of who we truly are, what we truly want and need. And we wonder why we feel so disoriented and tired to the core. We've given everything we have and have nothing left for us. Sound familiar?

When we're operating on a frazzled level, day-to-day, we're opening the door for so many illnesses to walk right in. We're creating the perfect storm for ill health – mental and physical.

But, to incorporate self-care into our everyday lives, we need to kick some existing habits to the kerb, introduce new ones and become mindful of what it is that truly makes us feel self-cared for. And that's no mean feat.

The very act of thinking about self-care can dredge up feelings of selfishness, guilt and unworthiness. We continue to put ourselves at the bottom of the list and wonder why we feel so frazzled, unfulfilled and antsy.

It's a minefield.

One we're going to face head-on.

Together.

This isn't any old book about self-care. The onus is on the word 'self' and what we might be able to learn about ourselves. In addition to my penny's worth, you will find journal prompts and suggestions of ways you can address some of the common barriers. Whether you decide to read it right through and then return to those, or pause when they arrive, it's up to you. Whatever feels right for you, is the name of the game.

Jayne x

PS. You can find me online – come and say 'hi':

[instagram] [twitter] @JayneHardy_

1. Who Am I to Write This Book?

'Self-care and I have a love–hate relationship.'

You're about to get acquainted with some of my foibles so to balance that out, I thought I'd kick things off with some notes of interest first. I'M really introverted – according to the Myers-Briggs personality test, I'm an INFJ. I've run two half marathons – the defining moment in one of those was being overtaken by a man dressed as a giant genital. My elbow joint is made from titanium and was shipped over from France – the result of a nasty (sober) tumble down the stairs as I was rushing to work one day. In nineteen eighty-something, I won Mini Majorette of the Year and was proper chuffed, chuffed enough about this particular achievement that it made it here, into this book. There's a rather fetching scar below my left eyebrow from a faceplanting incident when I was a tiddler – the toilet seat fared better than me. I married my sixth-form crush in Malta. I fell asleep mid-childbirth (too much diamorphine). I've flown a plane, done a bungee jump and been zorbing.

I am also a prolific ball juggler; I'm a mother, a wife, a daughter, a sister, a friend, a leader of a team, and can't have a shower without another 'good' idea popping into my head.

I bet you can guess which ball I drop the most frequently. Yep, you guessed it; the only ball I keep repeatedly dropping is the self-care ball – one of the most important balls of all. As an educated and (usually) rational human being, I have embarked on a quest to learn why that's the case. Why do I feel resistance to self-care? What is it about prioritising self-care that makes me feel so icky? And why, oh why, does it feel as though I self-sabotage anything that feels good for me? Why do I feel so darn undeserving?

I have a long history of depression, and my quest to get to grips with this self-care malarkey has often found me wondering which came first – my lack of self-care or my depression? It's a 'chicken or egg?' question, but science tells us that self-care and mental wellbeing are intrinsically linked.

Depression stole chunks of my life, leaving me unable to work, leave the house or undertake the most basic acts of self-care – losing a tooth because I didn't feel worthy enough to clean them. I felt exhausted, helpless and hopeless. I treated myself according to those thoughts.

Learning to manage depression only truly started when I reintroduced self-care. A practice that was totally at odds with how I was feeling. It hurt to be kind and caring with myself; it had become alien to treat myself so nicely.

'Learning to manage depression only truly started when I reintroduced self-care.'

It was my experience of depression – the isolation, the loss of hope and suicidal thoughts –

that led me to set up The Blurt Foundation in 2011.

I remember approaching my thirties and looking back over the past eight years. Depression had gobbled up most of my twenties, and I didn't want to lose another decade in the same way. I guess that was the point when I gave up giving up.

My self-care at this point was non-existent; I wasn't showering often nor eating properly. My hair was akin to a snake's wedding and although nobody ever told me, I must have smelled pretty revolting.

My bed was my safe place, and it was there that I hid from the world. Not realising at the time that, in seeking refuge, I was also creating a prison, of sorts, for myself. My window to the outside world was predominantly via social media. I could dip in and out when it suited me but also connect with people who were struggling in the same way I was. In fact, they were much braver than me because they were speaking about depression so candidly and without shame.

I was yet to reach that point.

Twitter also introduced me to blogging. I saw that there were people blogging about all sorts of things and I missed writing – it was something I'd always loved until depression sapped the joy and self-belief out of it for me. I decided that writing a beauty blog might help me with self-care. To write about beauty products I'd have to use beauty products – self-care, right there!

That little blog helped me in ways I'm not sure I can properly put into words; it gave me a purpose, distracted me from the suicidal thoughts, injected pleasure back into writing, brought some sunshine back into my life. I started taking better care of myself and seeing the glimmer of a future ahead.

The natural progression was to start writing about other things

'I strongly feel that nobody should go unheard and as such, we respond to every email and social media message.'

that were important to me.

I felt that as a beauty blog, it wasn't a very rounded view of what life was like for me at that time. I had an urge to write about depression but wasn't sure if I could or if I should.

I did end up writing a blog post about my experiences of depression. It was the very first time I tried to put it all into words, and it was a painful process – facing the dark when you're afraid of the dark always is.

That blog post changed everything.

Within twenty-four hours of publication, I received just over one hundred messages via email, text, Twitter, Facebook and blog comments. People I had known since primary school told me about their experiences of depression. I had no idea they were struggling too. Complete strangers thanked me for my honesty and for putting into words what they were experiencing.

Two things became crystal clear: 1) people were quite comfortable talking to me online, and 2) we were all struggling alone when we could be supporting one another.

And so, the idea for Blurt was born – a platform to kick-start conversations about depression, increase awareness and understanding, connect people, and reach them where they are (online). My experiences influence how we run Blurt as a social enterprise. I strongly feel that nobody should go unheard and as such, we respond to every email and social media message.

I also believe that to kick-start conversations; you need to speak to people in a friendly, informal and kind way. Internally, we place a huge focus on self-care and allow the team to work flexibly so that we minimise that work/life balance conflict as much as possible.

Our work with Blurt is only the tip of the iceberg regarding what needs to be done to help those affected by depression. Because of that, there's a tendency always to be looking ahead to see how we can reach and help more people. In doing so, it's easy to forget to stop and reflect on how much I have changed and how much, as a team, Blurt has achieved.

It's mind-boggling to me that we now have a team of thirteen people, that we had over two million page views on our website in 2016, that we receive letters, cards, emails and social media comments every day from people who say that we have helped them, that people credit us with saving their lives, and that every day we're witness to hundreds of people using their hindsight as another's foresight and support each other with such kindness, patience and generosity.

We truly listen to our audience; we consider them to be our stakeholders. The conversations we have with our audience shape our organisational priorities.

During those conversations, we also began to understand that the cultural emphasis on 'doing good' and 'giving, not taking' is putting pressure on people to be the 'doer of all things' and the 'taker of none'. It means we're depleted, never feel as though we're doing enough or being enough. We look at ourselves, see where we're lacking and spend the rest of the time making up for our shortcomings. Approval becomes external; we seek it from others, rather than

'Approval becomes external; we seek it from others, rather than seeking to approve of ourselves.'

seeking to approve of ourselves. Our kindness extends outwards, leaving very little, if any, for ourselves.

In October 2016, we launched the #365daysofselfcare challenge where we encouraged people to take part in a small act of self-care each day and to broadcast their efforts on social media. A few things became apparent: 1) people want to feel better, 2) they don't always understand what self-care means for them individually, and 3) guilt and resistance are to self-care what the Joker is to Batman.

And that's why I'm here, writing these words. We're going to drill down into the nitty-gritty, get to grips with why self-care is important, why it is that we struggle with it, and how to maintain a daily self-care habit.

You can find Blurt in these places:

Website: blurtitout.org
facebook.com/@blurtitout
@blurtalerts
@theblurtfoundation

We are all in this together and so it seems like a great idea to facilitate some hand-holding, connections, and pom-pom shaking across social media for the times we might run out of steam. We're using the hashtag #selfcareproject if you want to join us.

Nine Ways I've Sucked at Self-Care

Self-care and I have a love–hate relationship. I understand how important self-care is, I truly do, and when I incorporate self-care into my daily life, I reap the rewards tenfold. I'm a much better person for it. I love who self-care helps me become.

But, for reasons I am yet to fathom, I keep dropping the self-care ball as though it's a radioactive hot potato. I hate how difficult I find it to prioritise my needs, especially as I am so quick to encourage others to prioritise theirs. I hate the internal dialogue that takes place when I do take time out for me. The dialogue that sheds light on the things I 'should' be doing, people I 'could' be spending time with, the things that so-and-so 'would' do. You know, those 'coulda, shoulda, woulda' thoughts that we have on repeat like a broken record. Unfortunately, I don't think they go away either. We just get more resilient at ignoring them, better at carrying on regardless, and we fall head over heels in love with the results of our self-care shenanigans so that *not* doing them becomes more painful than doing them.

When it comes to the ways in which I have sucked at self-care, let me tell you, they're in plentiful supply – it took some savage shortlisting to include *just* nine ways I've sucked at self-care.

It feels important for me to talk about the times it's gone awry. We don't do that enough. We share our best bits willingly and with glee. We shout from the rooftops when things are going right for us, but we hide away when the going gets tough. Where are the examples of pain and rejection, the battles we've fought and lost, on our social media feeds? They're few and far between. But we all experience obstacles in life, and when we share the complicated mess of those, we open the door for others to do the same, which helps to diminish the shame we so often feel.

Nobody ever has their shizz completely together, despite how it might look from our ringside seats. We struggle, we experience heartbreak, things don't work out as we hoped and as we strive to grow into ourselves, that whole experience is an often-painful one. Growth hurts; it takes you on a journey through tough times and demands that you're self-aware enough to question everything inside and outside of you so that you can learn something along the way. When hope is fragile, and you're holding on by your fingertips, it takes buckets of courage to pick yourself back up again – and again, and again, and again, and again, and again.

Life *is* a rollercoaster, the lows somewhat more of an education than the highs. It's the lows that teach us valuable lessons and give us insights. They're where we get to grips with our true character and inner strength. That's something to be celebrated in ourselves and others; that we've experienced these terrific obstacles, navigated some prickly circumstances and made our way through them. The lows shouldn't be a source of malicious gossip and judgement, nor smugness. We're all just learning as we go.

I'm semi-proud of these moments I sucked at self-care. In knowing that I sucked, I have developed a self-awareness that allows me to see these incidences as they are. They're not episodes of failure, not sticks with which to beat myself, but times I might have taken better care of myself and should history repeat itself, I like to think that the outcome would be different. Where I'm still a work in progress, the self-awareness serves to hand me a list of self-care goals, a roadmap, if you like, of things I can improve upon with time. We only know what we know, and hindsight affords us the opportunity to reflect on circumstances knowing more today than we did back then. It's not an equal footing; we'll always look unfavourably at the things that didn't go so well because we're more informed now than we were then – we know how those decisions/actions played out.

With that in mind, I'm unashamedly sharing some cringeworthy truths with you.

1. A Year-Long Ear Infection

I've always had problems with my ears. If I'm a little run down, my ears and throat are the first to let me know. The hearing in my right ear is near non-existent due to countless ear infections I had as a child. You'd think then that I would be hugely respectful and thankful of the hearing in my left ear and would do whatever it took to protect its functionality so that I wouldn't be fully deaf. Makes sense, right? I agree, which is why this particular case of shoddy self-care confuses and bemuses me in equal measures.

In August 2015, my left ear started hurting and leaking some foul-smelling gunk. I went to the doctor and was given a course of antibiotics which reduced the pain but didn't make it go away, nor stop the yucky stuff from coming out of my ear. My hearing was also greatly reduced, which made conversing difficult – I just couldn't hear anyone particularly well. It affected my quality of life as I often didn't have the energy to concentrate on the conversations taking place around me – and I often felt as though I was a bystander, a bit left out, definitely an inconvenience when requesting that sentences were repeated, repeatedly. The pain was low level, definitely put-up-able, but it's anyone's guess why on earth I would choose to put up with it in the first place.

A year after that initial appointment, I went back to see my doctor. He prescribed an ear spray, and within forty-eight hours, my hearing was back, my ear had stopped leaking and the pain had gone.

2. Badger Hair

It's a sad fact of my life that, left to its own devices, my hair would have considerable grey coverage. The grey strands crept in when I was in my mid-twenties and have been spreading at a rate of knots ever since. As my hair dye grows out, I am left with a distinct badger stripe, which doesn't quite suit me – being a non-badger an' all. Taking that into consideration, I am yet to go and get my hair seen to in a timely manner. Emergency hair appointments are often made because I have an important meeting or event, never because it's just time to get it done. Never for my benefit. But you know what? As soon as I've been to that elusive hair appointment, I feel absolutely fantastic. It's a conundrum.

3. Going to University

I ended up at university because I hated my job, all my friends had disappeared to various university locations across the country and seemed to be having a whale of a time, and I just didn't know what I wanted to do or be. I was lost, bored and unfulfilled. Our school careers advice had consisted of two options: 1) to join the armed forces, or 2) to go to university. Having worked as a trainee accountant upon leaving sixth form and not at all enjoying it, going to university felt like the only option available to me. It was a rabid case of following the crowd and a gigantic mistake. I hated university; it just wasn't for me. Being away from home, the drinking culture, the boring course I'd chosen, the isolation, the lack of structure in the early weeks when I had only two hours of lectures, not quitting sooner than I did because I was embarrassed to return home as a 'dropout' . . . the list is endless.

4. Puke, Work, Puke, Work

When I was pregnant with our daughter, Peggy, I had hyperemesis gravidarum. HG is similar to morning sickness but all day, every day. I was vomiting, or feeling as though I was about to vomit, twenty-four hours a day. It was brutal. I lost 10 per cent of my body weight in those first twelve weeks of pregnancy and found myself in hospital hooked to a drip to get some fluids back into me. My kidneys were not in a good way, and neither was I. Thankfully, Baby Peggy was fine. Looking back, I'm incredulous that I didn't stop working throughout this. I worked between vomit breaks; I worked from my hospital bed. I just didn't stop. My health was in jeopardy, already Baby Peggy was incredibly precious to me, but still, I pushed my body to its limits. Nowt noble in that. Would do it all very differently if I had that time again.

5. I Don't Have a Dentist

At the age of eighteen, I found myself with a swollen and excruciatingly sore cheek. I ventured to the dentist to find that someone who had bullied me at school was now the dental assistant and on top of that I not only had an abscess which needed bursting, but I was also referred to the hospital to have all four wisdom teeth removed. Needless to say, it was a frightening experience, and I've not been back to see that dentist, or any other, since. Which leads me nicely on to . . .

6. Bye-Bye Molar

At the age of twenty-four, I found myself battling depression and slowly but surely, all self-care activities fell by the wayside. I wasn't eating properly, sleeping well or taking any notice of personal hygiene. I didn't feel worthy of the care, and the suicidal thoughts were telling me that there wasn't any point to it anyway, not for where I was heading. My teeth bore the brunt of this: a perfect teeth-ruination of no dental check-ups, no cleaning and a Diet Coke addiction led to me losing a molar as I bit into a slice of toasted granary bread. I didn't care at the time; I hardly

registered that it had happened but, as time goes on, I care more
and more and would like to get this, and my other tooth issues
(thank you, hyperemesis gravidarum) looked at.

7. Wonky Boundaries

This isn't a one-off occurrence for me – my boundaries are wonky
and asserting them feels icky. Often, my boundaries feel as
though they are a nuisance for others and this feeds right into
the low self-worth thing I'm working on. It also doesn't help
that I have empathy for those who are resisting my boundaries.
Their perspective on the situation makes sense to me; I
understand why they feel the way they feel and then I feel bad,
as though I am responsible. Rationally, I know that we're each
responsible for our own happiness, but if wonkifying a boundary
of mine makes life a little easier for someone else, you can bet
your last pound coin that I'll probably do it. I tend always to
regret it though and self-care for me, where boundaries are
concerned, is very much a work in progress, one that sees me
storing up responses to said boundary testing so that I am
prepared, but also feeling the fear and doing it anyway. It's also
about self-respect; we teach others to respect us by what we will,
and won't, allow. I would like my actions to speak louder than my
words so that my daughter grows up knowing this too.

8. All the Times I've Said 'Yes' When I Really Meant 'No'

This is a boundary issue in some parts but also feels different in many ways. I've never really felt as though I 'fit in' and as I grow older I am beginning to understand that's not such a bad thing. I'm growing more and more comfortable with my introverted quirky self, and that's nothing short of a revelation. But growing up, and at least until my early thirties, I so wanted to fit in; I was desperate to feel as though I 'belonged' somewhere. I would bend, twist and turn to do just that. It felt icky, I wasn't being at all authentic, I just wanted to be liked, and for that to happen, I thought I had to keep everyone happy. Other people's happiness became my benchmark. Talk about making a rod for your back. I became so attuned to reading others, to understanding what their needs, wants and expectations were, that I totally silenced my own. Doing so eventually came back to bite me on the bum. I wasted so much time and energy on doing things I really didn't want to do, which led to a right ol' muddle for me: resentment, trust issues, low self-esteem, seeking approval, giving so much of myself and losing my sense of self, to name a few. Not fun at all.

9. Custard Toupé, Anyone?

Parenthood simultaneously taught me that I would go to the end of the earth to make sure our daughter was happy and that to do so, I was going to have to take self-care waaaay more seriously. The parenting lessons came in thick and fast, but there's one incident that sticks in my mind – hindsight adds to its hilarity factor, alongside the lesson that when you're strung out, the little things are the big things (it's the straw that breaks the camel's back, after all).

Peggy was seven-ish days old, and we were yet to have a hot meal. Our world was in disarray as is always the way when you welcome something so tiny and dependent on you into your life. They say it takes a village to raise a child, but our village is more of a hamlet comprising very few people available to assist with child-rearing activities.

Baby blues were in full effect, the stitches 'down there' were getting on my wick, and in my post-hyperemesis gravidarum freedom, food had taken on a new level of joy. Tired, tearful and irrational, I wanted a hot meal, and it became the be all and end all. I wasn't alone – my husband was feeling pretty cranky and hankering after something warmer than a sandwich too, and so he cooked up a delicious meal with an apple crumble for dessert.

Peggy had been asleep whilst the food prep was underway; she started stirring as we were digging into our dinner, but we managed to get it down before our parental skills were needed. Except, I hadn't eaten my apple crumble and I *really* wanted to eat my apple crumble. Being all martyr-ish, I decided that it was only fair that Dom eat his in peace as he'd made it and that I would juggle baby and bowl. It'd be fine.

It wasn't fine.

A dollop of (cold) custard fell off my spoon and landed on Peggy's head. The mother of all meltdowns came next, and I don't think I even finished my crumble.

You'll be pleased to know that we've since become epic tag teamers and no crumble has gone uneaten.

Times I've sucked at self-care	What it taught me

Describe 10 interesting facts about YOU

1 _____

2 _____

3 _____

4 _____

5 _____

6 _____

7 _____

8 _____

9 _____

10 _____

What balls are you juggling?

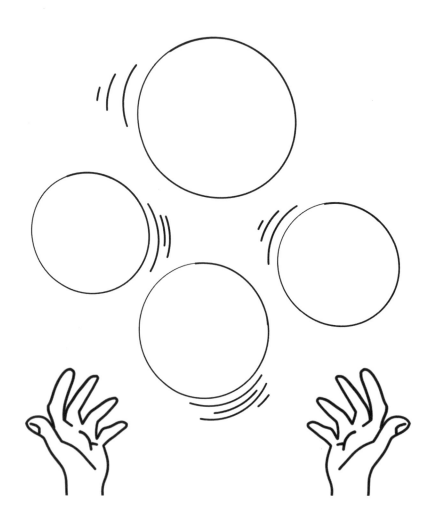

2. What is self-care?

'Despite what those pesky thoughts inside our heads tell us, self-care isn't selfish.'

If you think that self-care is the latest 'fad', 'trend' or 'buzzword', you're not alone. In recent years, the use of the term 'self-care' has been bandied about left, right and centre. It's very much 'on-trend' – there are over 44,600,000 results for the search term on Google. Everyone and their dog seem to be talking about it. We're being encouraged to take much better care of ourselves, by everyone and anyone.

But very much like mindfulness and gratitude, the teachings of self-care can be traced back in history. They're not new terms, teachings or concepts; they make complete and utter sense. More so now than ever: our lives are busy, and we're sick and tired of feeling sick and tired.

In fact, self-care has mindfulness as its foundation; you can't care for yourself in the truest sense if you don't understand what it is that you need, what it is that comforts you and nourishes you. Self-care requires you to become hyper-aware of how you feel all

'Our lives are busy, and we're sick and tired of feeling sick and tired.' day, every day. Being hyper-aware of how you feel then helps you to make choices based on those feelings. The right choices for you; what it is that you need to do to help you to feel good, both in the long term and the short term. We've all been there – we've agreed to do something for someone and instantly regretted it, leading to us feeling resentful and fraught. Instead of that simple 'no, sorry, I can't', we expend a tremendous amount of energy and headspace then trying to get out of it. In doing all of that, we've put that person's expectations/needs/wants/dreams/approval above our very own. We've prioritised that person and slowly slipped down the pecking order of what/who is important, often without even realising it.

Self-care is about taking responsibility for yourself. You're probably thinking, 'I already do!' And yes, you definitely do – whether that be to go to work, take care of a family, pay your bills or partake in a myriad of other 'adult responsibilities'. But self-care is about consciously taking responsibility for your happiness; your physical, emotional, psychological and social needs. And doing everything you can to ensure you feel fulfilled in those areas.

You partake in self-care without even knowing it; you wash, sleep and eat. But much of that happens on autopilot without a conscious sense of how it might be benefitting you. Are you getting enough sleep? Are you eating foods that nourish your body and your brain?

Only you will really know what self-care means for you. We're all different: our genetics, our experiences, our peer groups and our lifestyles. An activity that leaves one person feeling nourished could be the equivalent of walking on hot coals with bare feet and a blindfold for another.

To add to the confusion, as you grow and evolve as a person, what counts as self-care for you might evolve too. That's where the mindfulness comes in, helping you to keep up with your changing needs, wants and dreams.

And we're not keeping up with our needs, wants and dreams. We're not feeling happy, and we're not feeling well.

We've seen an astounding leap in technology in recent years and in many ways, that's a good thing – we can do our food shop from the comfort of our home (in our pyjamas, no less), we can pay all of our bills online (cheque books are pretty much obsolete nowadays), we can order gifts for friends to arrive at their homes the very next day (the same day, depending on where you live), some people don't even travel to work as technology allows them the option to work from home, and we can chat to people from all over the world, online.

Great stuff, right?

Yes, but all of that comes at a price.

Our lives are crammed full of activities – from the time we wake up until the moment we lay our heads on our pillows in the desperate hope for a good night's sleep. And we're still not getting it all done. We're at the mercy of our smartphones too, jumping when the flashing light or sound alert tells us to. There are a gazillion different ways we can be contacted, and we've got apps coming out of

'As you grow and evolve as a person, what counts as self-care for you might evolve too.'

our apps. We're stressed, frazzled, unfulfilled and overwhelmed. Happy? Who has time for happy? We'd love to partake in self-care but just don't have the time. We simply can't add another 'thing' to our already exhaustive list of 'things' to do. We're on the road to Sickville, and the worst thing is, we don't realise it until we arrive, depleted and unwell.

If we don't find the time for self-care, our health has a way of forcing us to stop and take care of ourselves somewhere down the line. If you don't find time to stop, your body and mind will force you to stop. And that's the truly scary bit. Because then, you have no other option but to prioritise self-care. That's, of course, if it isn't too late.

So much of the pressure we feel comes from living up to other people's expectations, their ideals and their needs/wants. They shout so loudly, and we get into the habit of serving them, to shut them up. We all like to be liked, but in serving other people's demands on our time and energy, we often end up silencing our individual needs and wants. We take responsibility for other people's happiness and forgo our own.

And that can't continue.

Despite what those pesky thoughts inside our heads tell us, self-care isn't selfish.

In fact, when we become self-care ninjas, we have so much more to give others. When we put our needs first, it often has a positive effect on the things that really matter to us – our health, our relationships, our resilience, our work. The people who have a problem with you taking care of yourself are the problem.

The ancient Greek philosopher Socrates understood the restorative power of self-care. He understood, too, the difference between self-care and self-interest. Two principles that are often confused.

There's a misconception in our modern times that putting ourselves first is an act of selfishness and that we should aim to be as selfless as possible – undermining the restorative power of self-care. Just as a motor vehicle can travel further when fuelled by a full tank of fuel – the correct fuel – we can give more, be more and help more when our tanks are full. Self-care allows us to be the very best version of ourselves, which in turn allows us to properly care for those around us. It facilitates our contribution to society in a way that aligns with our values (not because we feel we ought to, but because we have identified the things that matter to us, and want to help make a difference).

When we act from a place of self-interest, we're often focused on what we can 'have' rather than what we can 'be'. More often than not, we find ourselves in sticky situations which test our values to the max; motivated to 'keep up with the Joneses', placing more kudos on the letters after a person's name than who they are as a person, and focusing on short-term fulfilment at the expense of our long-term happiness.

Actions do speak louder than words, and when our actions are those of care, we show others how we would like to be treated but also teach them how to care for themselves.

This is what Socrates would refer to as the 'chain of care' – in practising self-care you teach others around you to do the same.

'Care of the soul' and 'know thyself' are believed to be the

'There's a misconception in our modern times that putting ourselves first is an act of selfishness.'

very first teachings about the concept of self-care as we know it today, and are woven throughout the 'Socratic way of life'.

Socrates lived between 470/469 and 399 BC. He has heavily influenced, through the works of Plato, Western culture and put his head above the parapet in his teachings of morals and ethics – very much against the beliefs and philosophies of his time. So much so that a jury of five hundred Athenians found him guilty of 'refusing to recognise the gods recognised by the state' and of 'corrupting the youth', and sentenced him to death for standing up for what he so passionately believed in.

Unfortunately, none of Socrates' original works exist; we only have secondary sources to rely upon, which is why we so often see him described as Platonic Socrates – through Plato's interpretation of Socrates' teachings.

Plato was another influential ancient Greek philosopher, thought to have lived between 428/427 and 348/347 BC. He was an innovative ol' chap too: he founded what is believed to be the very first university in the world – The Academy in Athens – where subjects such as biology, mathematics, astronomy, philosophy and political theory were taught. He was mentored, and inspired by Socrates, and went on to teach Aristotle (another of those incredible ancient Greek philosophers, who in turn went on to teach Alexander the Great, no less!). It is through the works of Plato that we are given an understanding of Socratic ethics and an insight into how to apply them in our modern-day lives.

In Plato's *Alcibiades I*, we first hear about 'care of self' (*epimeleia heautou*) in some detail. The term comes about when exploring the question, 'What is the self that the self must care for?' The answer: 'Taking care of oneself will be to take care of the self insofar as it is the "subject of" a certain number of things: the subject of instrumental action, of relationships with other people, of behaviour and attitudes in general, and the subject also of relationship to oneself.'

What this means is that when we take care of ourselves, we are embodying decisive and conscious action. Self-care also includes the relationships we have with other people (and our boundaries within those relationships), behaving in a way that aligns with who we truly are and treating ourselves with the attention, kindness and respect we deserve.

It is also in Plato's *Alcibiades I* that Socrates builds the case for the importance of self-knowledge. There is a famous inscription on the wall of the Temple of Apollo at Delphi, which says *'gnōthi seautón'* – know thyself.

It is only in knowing ourselves that we can care for ourselves effectively. We need to know who we are – our principles, values, ethics and morals – establish our boundaries and explore how certain decisions and activities make us feel, and then be disciplined to discover why we may feel or react in that way.

And, at times, our truth will contradict what we've come to know about ourselves, or what we feel to be our obligations. It might (and probably will) differ from the distracting 'truths' we are fed by the media and the world at large.

There will also be times where our truth will shed light on some home truths; things which may cause us pain or discomfort, or lead us to feel unsettled by their discovery; we may unwrap resentment towards certain people in our lives, discover that we don't particularly enjoy our jobs or expend energy and time on people we really don't want to. Nobody said this self-care malarkey was going to be easy!

According to Socrates, 'care of self' and to 'know thyself' are fundamental principles regarding the healthy relationship we have with ourselves, and others. In taking care of ourselves and knowing ourselves, we reduce the risk of harming others because we become more aware of our boundaries, means and potential. He believed that knowing ourselves allows us to save ourselves and to explore new approaches to living.

It's not an angle that we often consider, but by not partaking in self-care, we are partaking in self-neglect, as passive as that may be. The scary thing is that we don't mean to neglect our needs, but we do so all the same. We're not committing to ourselves in the short term and long term, which can only lead to one thing – we're cruising down the highway to catastrophe for our health: mental and physical.

The lines between commitment, hard work and self-neglect are often so blurred that it becomes commendable – exhaustion a badge of honour, an 'in joke' with our peers. We become so concerned about fitting in, achieving, having the approval of others, being all things to all people, that we set about destroying ourselves in the process. And yes, it does sound a bit dramatic, doesn't it?!

But consider the benefits of brushing our teeth: good oral hygiene prevents tooth decay, gum disease, bad breath, oral cancer and costly dental fees. A relatively simple act of personal hygiene prevents all that ill health.

'It is only in knowing ourselves that we can care for ourselves effectively.'

Self-care prevents disease. It's the best preventative measure available to us. To make the best possible use of it, we need to heighten our self-awareness, self-monitoring and self-reflection skills, and honour our findings. Change our perspective on the way we lead our lives. Understand that above all else in importance are our physical, emotional, psychological and social needs. We begin by paying heed to the often subtle signs that tell us to step back, to stop, to flex.

'There's no denying that the key to optimum health and happiness lies in self-care.'

And the early warning signs are *always* there – we just don't take notice: exhaustion, niggly aches and pains, lumps and bumps, lack of motivation and feeling overwhelmed, to name a few. Rather than explore them to get to the root of their cause, we ignore them and keep on trucking on, placing our minds, our organs and our relationships under incredible stress. According to the European Health Parliament, a lowly 3 per cent of health budgets are earmarked for ill health prevention activities, which means we need to take the baton, take responsibility for our health and wellbeing. Nobody else will.

There's no denying that the key to optimum health and happiness lies in self-care.

We're rarely at the top of the pecking order, where we belong. Where do you feel you're currently at?

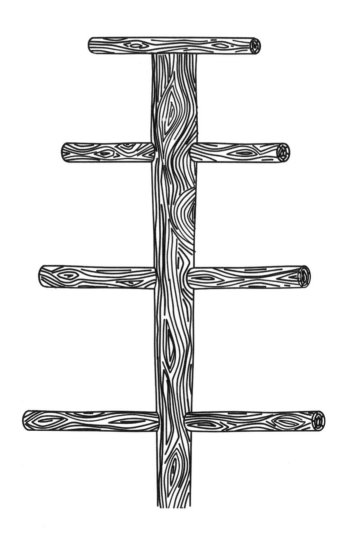

Use the gauge below to mark how full
or un-full your tank is right now.

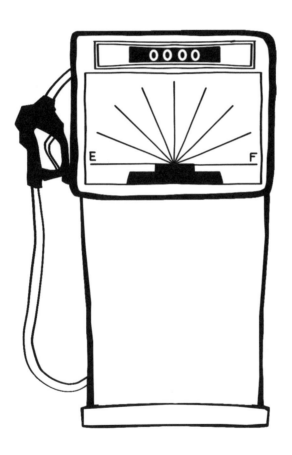

This is a monthly mood tracker. Decide on differing moods for your colour-coded key and fill in an area of the fish a day, to represent the mood which summed up the day for you.

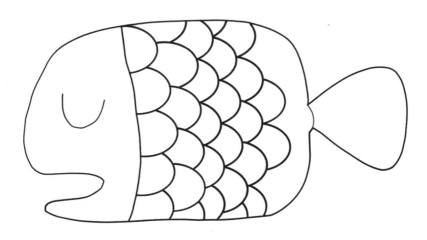

Mood key

☐ eg. calm   ☐   ☐

☐   ☐   ☐

3. Why self-care is important

'The manner of self-care is that it spurs us to foster connections with ourselves first and foremost.'

The term 'self-care' often conjures up a myriad of fluffy scenes; a steaming hot bubble bath with scented candles burning away, a trip to a countryside beauty spa, a romantic candlelit dinner, perfectly manicured and pedicured digits, luxury face masks, pool-side holidays, Instagram-able adventures, picnics in the park with good friends, a cosy night in . . .

And those things *are* examples of self-care, for sure – for some. They're just not the whole picture. Those scenes make self-care seem as though it's an elusive club for the wealthy and time-rich. They're grand-ish gestures, treats, if you will, not things that we could easily build into our everyday lives. In the scheme of life, they're not realistic self-care practices to strive for and if they're what we think self-care is, in its entirety, then the very notion of this 'out of reach' version of self-care can lead us to feel despondent and powerless. It becomes easier to explain it away; it validates those 'it's not for people like me' suspicions we may harbour. You see, the truth about self-care is that it's nearly always *not* fluffy; it can be downright boring. But don't be fooled – being boring doesn't diminish its importance nor its epic transformational abilities. Boring self-care might include making that overdue doctor's appointment, getting enough sleep, remembering to take your meds, calling a crisis team, brushing your teeth, tidying your home, sorting through your finances, applying for a job, eating a nutritious meal, arranging childcare, completing forms, making an uncomfortable telephone call, doing the laundry, taking a shower, asserting your boundaries, asking for help, etc. The seemingly dull nature of these activities we call 'life admin' often means we procastinate over them or avoid them altogether, but their very nature means they often act as preventative measures. When we neglect 'life admin' for a sustained period of time, we increase the risk of turbulence in our lives. Turbulence that ends up being much more difficult to deal with than the tasks would originally have been.

Everything that exists in our lives is the result of a set of decisions, choices and actions. Everything. The scary thing about that is we can get caught up in the minutiae, routine and external pressure, which means we end up with results that aren't aligned with our wants and needs. That has a massive psychological and emotional impact on us. To arrive at an outcome (be it one we've consciously chosen or one we're heading towards without realising) we tend to follow a process; a process of microscopic actions and decisions which are usually a little lacklustre in isolation. It's on the continuum of a series of lacklustre actions and decisions, which are aligned with a consciously set goal, where the extraordinary lives. The devil is in the detail. It helps us tremendously to know what we want to be/do/feel because it affords us the chance to reverse engineer that outcome and provides us with a blueprint of the steps we need to take to get there.

Consider the excitement you feel about going on holiday and the steps you might need to actually get there – some kind of financial audit might be required in order to put away some savings, the completion of a passport form is often an arduous one, the timeframe a tricky navigation, choosing where to go and with whom, completing annual leave request forms with your employer, possibly a visit to the doctor to have some jabs, insurance quotes to trek through and pay for, parking charges to pay, packing – the list of things you need to do to actually get to the point where you arrive at your holiday destination is a long one. And cumbersome. But because you have made a conscious decision that this holiday is something you're committed to – it's exactly where you want to end up – the steps you need to take to get there become clearer. You're willing to go through the boring process because the result is well worth it.

Self-care is no different. The steps might not be attractive in their isolation but if we know where we want to be, who we want to be, how we want to feel and what we want to do, self-care is just a term for the process of helping us get from A to B. This *knowing* is the tool that guides us to make better, educated, thoughtful and proactive decisions. If that's not enough to get your head around, in addition to the 'fluffy' assumptions, the term 'self-care' tends to be an emotive one – it makes us 'feel' something. Whether that 'something' is that you feel selfish or perhaps self-indulgent even *considering* prioritising your needs, or you experience shame that you can't afford those fluffy things, or you're annoyed by the seeming flippancy of it all, or worried that it may appear that you can't cope. The term might set off a bout of comparisonitis, prompt an 'eye roll' as you're fed up with hearing about it – it's everywhere and has lost its meaning for you – or perhaps you are spinning so many plates in the air that you're too overwhelmed to even stop and consider what self-care means for you. There's a recurrent resistance that we feel to self-care.

Isn't that the stickler for so many of us when self-care is on the table?

It's a loaded subject because to give it a go, we need to consider ourselves a priority and we just don't see ourselves in that way. To give it our best shot, we need to also consider our vulnerabilities and we just don't *want* to see ourselves in that way, either – it makes us feel naked, exposed.

We're taught empathy, consideration and understanding of others, to help, to contribute, to work hard . . . but we're rarely taught about our individual emotional and psychological make-up. That does us all a disservice.

The word 'self' can instigate that ants-in-your-pants cringe-shuffle (you totally know the one!) on a par with the awkwardness we feel when complimented. Being asked to put ourselves first is often an icky proposition. We're uncomfortable. The thoughts conflict. Perceptions conflict. Life is hectic enough as it is. Our minds are full. Our hands are full.

To add salt to the wound, we ignore the inkling that something isn't working for us. That this hamster wheel version of life that we're living can't continue. There's a gnawing feeling in the pit of our stomachs that urges us to take stock but we don't

'To give it our best shot, we need to also consider our vulnerabilities.'

pay heed to it. Our priorities are swallowed up by the ideals and expectations of others, and scarily, we keep ploughing on until our health or other circumstances force us to stop.

'Change is hard. It's unsettling. It's painful.'

We're not necessarily disgruntled with every aspect of our lives, either. It's possible to simultaneously feel grateful and dissatisfied, motivated and scared, exhausted and hopeful. We don't belong in boxes with labels, we're naturally complex and contradictory creatures.

Change is hard. It's unsettling. It's painful.

But when our unhealthy habits are prolonged, change will always become unavoidable. Either we lead the proactive charge or we wait until the day our hand is forced.

Rock. Hard place.

As a species, it doesn't help that we're not mighty fans of change. Yes, it's a natural progression of life and on a physical level, our bodies are constantly renewing and changing as we age. But mentally, comfort is found in the habitual. Change often means that something is coming to an end. And we should allow the space to grieve that ending, no matter what it is that's ended.

We understand that things do, and need to, change. But to actively bring about the process of change? No thanks, we'd rather avoid it. Change brings with it fear of the unknown, fear of failing, self-doubt, resistance from others, renewed effort, the need to challenge existing perceptions and to root through our emotional baggage. We'd much prefer to remain in our comfort zones where we feel safe, in control and at ease.

How often, too, have we heard the phrase 'hasn't she/he changed?!'

bandied about as though it's a negative thing? We don't feel comfortable when we've activated the change and we most certainly don't feel comfortable when those around us change, either.

Then we have the catalysts for change that usually mean we're already not operating from the best place. The circumstances that prompt or demand change can be painful in themselves. And whilst breakdown often breeds breakthrough, that's a sucky starting point if ever there was one.

The manner of self-care is that it spurs us to foster connections with ourselves first and foremost, to make tweaks, to flex and to review aspects of our lives on a day-by-day basis. It calls for us to sit up and to be mindful in all that we do. To trust ourselves. To give ourselves permission to go all in, to be happy. To question the 'why' behind our actions. To understand that we are enough, with all our glorious quirks. To monitor how we feel and look for patterns in the good and bad. To make changes as we go, long before breakdown occurs. To face problems head on and to promptly seek their solutions. There are a gazillion reasons why we resist change, yet one strong reason to embrace it – the promise of a better feel for life. The lure of good health, vitality and happiness. Those are the things we compromise when we deny ourselves the opportunity to change things up.

For self-care to be effective, for it to be as transformative as it can potentially be, we need to take a long hard look in the mirror and really get comfortable with who we are, warts an' all. Not only is that period of discovery going to be an additional task on top of our already hectic lives, it's going to be an ongoing process which isn't always a comfortable one. No wonder we avoid it like the plague.

Our individuality is the thing we all have in common. Heritage, genetics, experiences and personality mean that we're all unique. Yet we find it difficult to embrace our 'us-ness', compromising who we are to fit in with the ideals and expectations of others.

Akin to the terms 'self-care' and 'mindfulness', the term 'authentic' is another gem that's been used so often that it no longer seems to hold any weight. Authenticity doesn't stem from our social status, awards and achievements but from embracing our originality, being genuine and living purposefully. Not from bending and weaving to 'fit in' but from understanding who we are, our essence as human beings. When we compromise our sense of self (and we all know when we're doing this as it makes us feel out of sorts) it erodes our self-esteem and self-confidence.

For us to be 'real' in the way we interact with others, in how we hold ourselves accountable, in how we make decisions and adhere to our code of conduct, in whether we permit ourselves to be who we really are, we need to *know* who we really are. This allows us to narrow the gap between who we are on the inside and what we present to the world. We can't answer questions, even simple questions such as 'what would you like to drink?' effectively and truthfully, unless we know ourselves well enough to answer honestly. And crucially, we need to step up and be brave enough to answer the questions with honesty. Think about it – do we really want a cup of tea 'as it comes'? Allowing others to decipher our ambiguous answers means we could literally end up with anything. We've just given away our power and placed ourselves at their mercy, not knowing where that leads.

We need to take time to drill down into the nitty-gritty of who we are:

What are our gripes?

Our strengths, our weaknesses?

What do we fear?

What are our dreams?

What are our boundaries, our limitations?

Where do we stand morally on certain topics?

What's our code of conduct?

What holds us back?

What energises us?

What drains us?

It takes courage to delve this deeply; we're not always going to like what we find. And that's okay because we're going to learn more about our weaknesses – the not-so-pleasant bits – but also discover more about our strengths.

Satisfaction doesn't come from moseying through life, reacting to external factors, feeling trapped and getting stuck in ruts with habits that no longer serve us.

We exist in a world where we're living to deadlines set by others; social interactions are plentiful but not necessarily of any meaning; we have a revolving to-do list which seems to grow quicker than the rate at which we can cross items off; and we want to be great at everything *now* – there's no room for error or progress. We've become prolific multi-taskers, rushing from one job to another without pausing for breath. And we're competitive too, thanks to social media. Our days are crammed to the brim because that's the only way we feel we can keep afloat of all the pressure.

We chase balance but we don't typically find it because there is no 'balance' to be found, no happy medium. We tend to compromise ourselves on the whimsical quest to achieve something that doesn't exist. Life doesn't allow for all our ducks to be perfectly lined up in a row. When we cast our focus on something, it means we're often sacrificing something else. Unfortunately, that sacrifice is often ourselves. And we don't even realise we're doing it.

Self-care, with all its fluffy first impressions, is far from fluffy. It's a mighty tool. When we take it seriously, even with the shakiest of commitments, it works hard for us. It underpins all that we do, it helps us to be the best version of ourselves, it benefits our mental and physical health, reduces the risk of burnout, helps us to perform better in all areas of our lives, to love wholly, to sustain ourselves, to have energy, clarity and focus.

It's a short- and long-term approach that allows you to be the captain of your own ship.

The Self-Care Alarm Bells We So Often Ignore

We're all living and breathing proof that miracles do exist. The odds of our conception are mind-bogglingly low. That, in and of itself, is pretty darn amazing, don't you think? Let that sink in for a moment – you're a miracle. Yup, YOU. You might not feel like one but science states that the chances of you being here are nothing short of miraculous.

Since the very moment you became a 'being', every cell of you has worked hard with very little conscious input or effort from you. These humble cells have protected, renewed, restored, regenerated, cleaned, circulated, eliminated, and kept you alive. They care for you every millisecond of every day, without a break, and we're not as appreciative of this as we could be.

We're finely tuned, complicated machines and where self-care is concerned, it helps to think of ourselves as just that – machines. Not in a robotic sense as though we have a part in an Arnold Schwarzenegger movie, but instead in the sense that our organs have mechanical functions which need servicing and maintaining, and which let us know, albeit in often subtle ways, when something isn't performing as it should. To work at our optimum, we also need to consider our input, what we demand of those working parts and how we might take them for granted.

Self-care is often used as an emergency measure to rebuild the damage, mentally and/or physically, that has already been done. We wait until we are unwell before we take it seriously and use self-care as a rehabilitation measure, only to stop those restorative habits when we're back up and running. We don't consider that self-care can also be used as a preventative measure to ease any pressure we might be feeling on a rolling basis. We adopt the irrational logic of wishful thinking that these niggles, aches, pains and unease will disappear of their own accord. We deny and downplay their existence, underestimate their seriousness, shrug them off as we don't like to make a fuss or trouble others, and feel we ought to be able to cope with whatever life throws our way. We certainly don't listen to them, nor accommodate them – we're too busy for that, thank you very much!

We'd make life so much easier for ourselves if we were to listen to our internal communication system – it's smart, it knows our bodies better than we do, and it works on a need-to-know basis, only nudging you to take better care of your body when you really need to do just that. You've most certainly felt your internal communication system in action too; sweaty palms when you're nervous, hunger pangs, thirst, a feverish high temperature.

It's true that the outside word is a deafening one and that tuning out that noise so that we can listen to the signals our bodies are attempting to bring to our consciousness is a skill we need to master. When we do listen to those ever-so-subtle cues and heed their message, we can act quickly and often minimise, if not eradicate, any damage to ourselves.

Those 'cues' act as alarm bells asking us to stop, slow down, listen, and tweak our self-care accordingly. We frequently override these subtle signals, which puts us more and more out of touch with ourselves. We're scared to stop because we're struggling to handle our caseload even when we're operating at full capacity. Our lives are so full that we don't often hear those alarm bells until they're so blindingly obvious that we have no choice but to stop and listen. If you put anything under prolonged stress, it will break. Our minds and bodies are no exception.

Inability to Switch Off

When our brains just won't stop with their planning, plotting, worry and problem solving, it's often a sign that we've been overdoing things and might not be giving ourselves enough of a break. Our brain needs space to digest the day and then it will cleverly work through the events and file them away for later use. When we don't give the brain a chance to rest, it never quite catches up and we feel 'wired', as though we have too many tabs open; we might experience restlessness when awake, yet have fitful sleep and never feel rested upon waking. With the bombardment of technology and information, we're digesting more data than ever before, putting our brains, and health, under strain. We can counter this by taking our full lunch hour (preferably away from our desk), building in regular pauses to our day, unplugging from technology, taking our full annual leave, prioritising leisure time, getting enough sleep and silencing alerts on our smartphone: all of which help to slow the pace.

'Our brain needs space to digest the day.'

We're Overwhelmed

When the world feels intimidatingly loud and as though it's closing in on us, everything feels as if it's a bit much to handle, we're dropping balls left, right and centre, or we start fantasising about escaping or evading our lives, that's the point we need to regroup, prioritise, rest, ask for help, say 'no', delegate and stop. They're classic signs that you're under considerable stress, that life has gone a bit topsy-turvy and some adjustments are needed.

Being Prickly

We've all been there – at that point where everything feels irritating and frustrating. We snap at others, feel affronted by the smallest of things, lose our sense of humour, and everything feels as though it's working against us. Life is pelting lemons our way and we handle it with the tactility of a cactus. We start to feel as though it's the world versus us and it gets our back up. Our prickly nature prevents anyone getting close enough to comfort and reassure, making us an island. Arguments and petty disagreements feature heavily during this time of prickliness, adding to the irritation and frustration. We know we're stepping out of line and we're not proud of it. It's hard to see the wood for the trees when all that's in front of you is problem after problem, challenge after challenge, and you're tired to your core. No man is an island and there are times when we need a break, we need help and we need encouragement. Allow others close enough to offer those things and remember, you can and will get through this.

Aches and Pains, Lumps and Bumps

Perhaps the loudest of all alarm bells we ignore. It's not normal to hurt, unless there's an explanation such as a heavy gym session, a half-marathon endeavour or a Ben Nevis expedition – and even then, pain will be relative. It's not normal to have lumps and bumps where there was nothing but smoothness before.
These are physical alarm bells of foghorn volume which require medical attention. And soon. *Yesterday* soon.

Cancelling Plans

We're not talking about the cancellation of plans that it makes good sense to cancel – the ones we really didn't want to commit to in the first place or the ones we've had a change of heart about. It's the cancellation of plans where we would find them downright enjoyable or where we're playing dodgeball with those important medical appointments that are a worry. They're a worry because they're a sign that we're putting ourselves at the very bottom of the scrapheap and choosing instead to react to demands placed on us by others. It's important to make time for ourselves as it pays dividends to do so. It helps to make a list of 'non-negotiables' – the things that are of the utmost importance for self-care – and asking for help from others to keep you accountable.

Loneliness

According to Maslow's 'hierarchy of needs', 'belongingness' is one of our five basic needs: we're wired to be social; we *need* intimate relationships and to feel as though we belong and are accepted. When there's an absence of love and connection, we are susceptible to loneliness.

It's the irony of the times we live in that, with all the gadgets we have at our disposal, we're lonelier than ever before. We're hyper-connected but those connections can be superficial and don't always meet our basic needs.

Loneliness affects the same part of our brains that physical pain does and has considerable health implications: it causes a raise in the body's stress response, suppresses the immune system, affects the blood flow to organs, increases our risk of morbidity and raises blood pressure.

For relationships to thrive, we need to prioritise time to maintain and foster them. If we're experiencing loneliness then we need to commit more time to relationships, otherwise we're jeopardising our health.

Irrational Behaviour

To remain conscious and mindful of our decisions and actions takes concentration, focus and energy. But when our brains have had enough, the self-control and self-discipline we usually master have eaten up the limited supply. We all have occasions when we indulge in impulsive behaviour, take more risks, act out of character and do things that don't seem to make any sense, to us or those around us. This is usually a sign of exhaustion. We're depleted. It's time to take a step back and take some time out for yourself.

I want to do, be, have and feel

- ○
- ○
- ○
- ○
- ○
- ○
- ○
- ○
- ○
- ○
- ○
- ○

- ○
- ○
- ○
- ○
- ○
- ○
- ○
- ○
- ○
- ○
- ○
- ○

Make a playlist of songs which inspire, uplift and make you smile

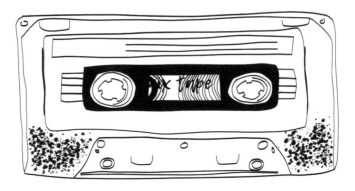

1
2
3
4
5
6
7
8
9
10

Pop your favourite quote/mantra in here

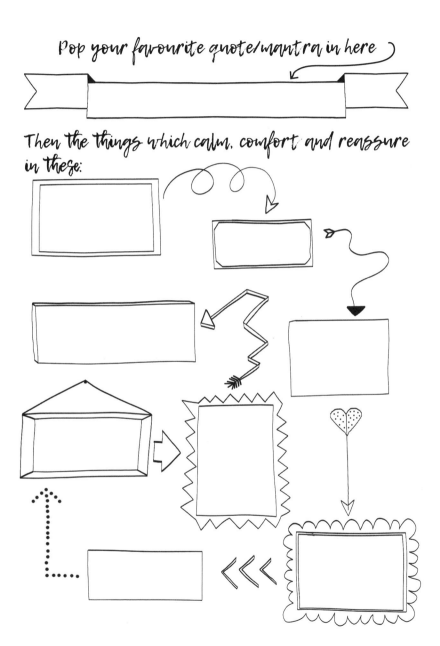

Then the things which calm, comfort and reassure in these:

4. The things that get in our way

'Barriers to self-care come at us from all directions; life is like a real-time, non-stop Tough Mudder circuit.'

It's one thing understanding that self-care makes sense and another to feel as though it's achievable. Life can often feel like we're on a real-life set of Mario Kart with obstacles coming at us thick and fast. It's how we 'see' those obstacles that will affect whether or not we'll make the changes we've identified that we'd like to make.

We may hold the view that those obstacles are roadblocks that derail us completely; that overcoming them is impossible, outside our remit. Or, we may view them as challenges and delve inside ourselves to come up with a solution to help us to overcome them, having the belief that we can do just that.

Our approach is down to our mindset and our mindsets are powerful ol' beasts – they dictate how we view ourselves and the world around us, and they shape our behaviours and our attitudes.

'Your mistakes are your lessons; you analyse the mistake and learn from it.'

According to Carol Dweck, an esteemed psychologist from

Stanford University, there are two types of mindset: a growth mindset and a fixed mindset.

'We do the best we can, with what we know.'

You have a fixed mindset if you are rigid in your thoughts. You believe, one way or another, that you can or can't achieve something and there's no leeway. You may feel ashamed of mistakes, scared of failure, fearful of challenges, and believe that any abilities you have, you were born with. The negative self-talk is brutal and centred on your perceived shortcomings. You may feel powerless, at the mercy of the world around you, and often a bit 'stuck'.

You have a growth mindset if you believe that you're a work in progress and love learning new things. Your mistakes are your lessons; you analyse the mistake and learn from it. You're aware of your strengths and weaknesses but not limited by them, understanding that you can build on the strengths and improve the weaknesses. You work hard to be who you want to be and to achieve your goals. You're resilient, tenacious and not afraid of challenges – you expect that they'll feature in life and you welcome the lesson within them.

These mindsets are interchangeable – you can work to shift from one outlook to another.

Both mindsets will approach these self-care shenanigans in different ways. A person with a growth mindset might relish the chance to learn something new; they'll be likely to feel motivated to tweak their lives to make sure there's time for self-care and certainly not think twice about dropping any habits that don't serve them. A person with a fixed mindset might write self-care off as something they just don't have time for, nor the abilities required to master it.

It's easy to read this and cast judgements. The growth mindset does have a desirability factor; it sounds more fun, empowering and liberating. Sexy, even. Yet,
so many of us don't live with that mindset.
We have a fixed mindset and the very nature of that mindset means that we're stumped, at a loss of what to do and how to do it. Our self-belief has done a runner and we feel a bit conked out with the exhaustion of it all. Putting ourselves 'out there' with no certainty of the outcome feels a stretch too far.

The exhaustion we feel is largely down to the emotional baggage we carry. It weighs us down and alters our perception. Emotional baggage isn't something we are born with. Certainly, we may be born into circumstances that don't nurture our emotional intelligence, but as newborn babies we just don't have the capacity to store conscious memories yet.

Life happens.

There is no script to life, no handbook to guide the way. We're on a parallel with others, venturing into the unknown. It's very much a process of trial and error, building our backstory as we go.
It's rich with experiences; some good, some bad and some downright ugly ones. We do the best we can, with what we know, having been influenced by our caregivers, our teacher and our peers. It's a mishmash, a tapestry, and quite frankly it doesn't always make any sense.

The hope for anyone would be that throughout life we are emotionally supported in such a way that we can deal with painful experiences as and when they happen: traumatic times, harmful interactions, mistakes we make, people who've misunderstood us, people we've misunderstood, rejection and heartache. But that's not always the case. When we don't receive emotional support, when we aren't taught about emotional tools, those painful experiences are hard to resolve and so they mould us and affect our ongoing behaviour.

Our emotional baggage is a culmination of all those negative experiences. They weigh heavy, that's for sure. We all have *some* sort of baggage; residue from our past experiences. The trouble with baggage, though – whether it's a bumbag or a giant suitcase – is that it affects everything: the relationships we have with others, the relationship we have with ourselves, how we see ourselves, how we see others, our thoughts, our decisions, our actions.

When we carry anything for too long, it takes its toll on our physical and mental wellbeing. It becomes heavier over time. The baggage might manifest in our current lives as: low self-worth, low self-confidence, self-sabotage, trust issues, commitment issues, avoidance, unease, feeling like an imposter, exhaustion, fear, shame, anger, resentment, negative self-talk and/or envy.

Emotional baggage is quite literally the feeling that you're carrying the weight of the world on your back.

Dealing with that baggage is never going to be a quick or easy task. It can be nothing short of terrifying to open that 'can of worms' and have to deal with the messy and complicated fallout. It's only by having a root through and putting some of those experiences to bed that we're able to move past them.

Our emotional baggage isn't the only thing that can hold us back, nor the only thorn in our side. We may, at times, find ourselves in the middle of some self-defeating behavioural shenanigans. When our actions aren't aligned with our desired

'Self-care is the opportunity to refuel so that we can give more to the world outside us.' outcome of a situation, one that's within our ability and control, then there is probably some self-sabotage at work; the instances when we make things difficult for ourselves. We get in our own way.

We don't half give ourselves a hard time, but others can give us a hard time too. Barriers to self-care come at us from all directions; life is like a real-time, non-stop Tough Mudder circuit. Navigable as long as we know what to prepare for.

Guilt

There's no sinking-sand feeling quite like the way we feel buried beneath guilt, layered upon guilt, layered upon guilt, layered upon some more guilt, with a big dollop of guilt on top for good measure.

Guilt is the biggest obstacle we face when self-care is on the table and the reason we find it so hard to prioritise our needs. We feel guilty for everything: for what we do, what we didn't do, for who we are, for who we aren't. We feel guilty for feeling guilty. The guilt is rampant and it keeps us in limbo.

When we feel guilty, it's usually because we are living according to the 'Law of Should'. The Law of Should has been dictated by society, by anyone other than ourselves really, and its legislation is bursting with expectations about how we 'should' lead our lives; how we 'should' parent, how clean our homes 'should' be, how much exercise we 'should' do, the foods we 'should' eat, the qualifications we 'should' aim for, the places we 'should' live, the hours we 'should' work, how we 'should' look and how we 'should' feel.

The Law of Should expects nothing short of perfection and we all know that there's no such thing. Which means that by living according to this law, we're chasing our tails, living according to a ridiculous collection of rules made by others. It leaves no room for anything other than self-judgement, self-criticism and guilt. It undermines our own authority to make choices and leads to a whole lorry-load of guilt.

We can't be everything to everyone. We just can't. Especially when we don't allow space for self-care. Self-care isn't a guilty pleasure; it's neither indulgent nor selfish. The guilt tells us that we're doing something wrong by prioritising our needs. But self-care is the opportunity to refuel so that we can give more to the world outside us. It sets a good example to those around us, giving them permission by proxy to do the same. There's nothing honourable about having to drag ourselves through each day, in being so depleted that we have nothing left to give. In fact, that's a pretty painful place to be. We don't want to ever end up there.

Not Asking for Help

As babies, we don't hesitate to ask for help. We wail loudly until we get it. It's a primitive, instinctive, inbuilt mechanism for survival and it works. As we grow older, it's not so black and white. There's a fine line we tread between growing in independence and knowing

'Asking for help needn't be a source of shame.'

when to ask for help. We judge ourselves for needing help; we perceive it as a character flaw, evidence of our weaknesses.

We worry that we'll be a burden, we worry that the person won't care enough to help, we feel as though we don't deserve that help, as though we haven't earned it, as though it's in limited supply. When we're offered help, we doubt the sincerity, we treat it as a token gesture.

But we're not designed to be a self-sufficient species; we flourish with meaningful connections with others and work well in teams. The fastest way to deepen and strengthen our relationships is to share our experiences, all of them. Not just our best bits, where we shine brightly, but also the unpleasant ones, which call for us to swallow our pride, shame, humility and vulnerability.

The anomaly is that we're keen to help others; we hate to think that someone is suffering alone, that they're too scared to turn to us for help.

The rules change depending on our stance; whether we're the person in need or the helper.

From time to time, we need help. It's a fact of life – we only know what we know and there will be moments when we need some assistance to help us fill in the gaps of our knowledge or to walk with us through the darkest of days. When someone calls on our support, it allows us an opportunity to make a difference, to use our hindsight as their foresight, to show we care. It's not a one-way exchange – both parties benefit from it.

At points, we'll need to call in reinforcements, by way of professional help, to support us as we navigate through the painful memories, thoughts and feelings in a safe way. That's what those services are there for: to be used.

Asking for help needn't be a source of shame. Doing so earlier rather than later prevents the problem from escalating into something bigger. You'd help others if they were to ask you; don't be afraid to reach out too.

Not Helping Ourselves

We treat others with way more respect and kindness than we treat ourselves. Way more. We'd never get away with treating others in the same shoddy and demeaning way that we treat ourselves.

Each person has a running commentary; non-stop mental chat that's relentless and domineering in nature.

The tone of this chit-chat matters. It's important. The way we speak to ourselves affects our view of our abilities. By putting ourselves down 24/7, judging ourselves harshly and belittling ourselves, we are taking a very bleak view of who we are. We gradually put others on a pedestal and we just don't match up. It's not a fair comparison; we have misted-up grey-tinted spectacles on to look inward and we replace them with sparkly rose-tinted ones when considering the attributes of others. The best-laid intentions for self-care never materialise as we over-accommodate the needs and whims of others because we see them as better than us, worthier. We write off our hard-earned achievements to luck, we start feeling as though we are severely lacking, that we're not good enough. Before we know it, we've become our own worst enemies.

There's a massive difference between being self-aware about why we made a mistake, learning from it and taking a different approach next time, to using our mistakes as a stick with which to beat ourselves. In small doses, self-criticism isn't a bad thing – it can motivate us to go get 'em (whatever those goals and dreams might be) – but if you tell anyone something repeatedly, they'll start to believe it. Relentless nasty self-talk causes us harm.

Nothing will bloom in such a bleak and destructive environment.

Decision Avoidance

We live in a choice-rich world. There are options aplenty, which require mental analysis before we can arrive at a decision. Even the trivial decisions follow this process. With so many decisions to make, is it any wonder that making them gets tiresome? Everything we do takes a decision of sorts and we find ourselves with decisions on top of our decisions.

Decision fatigue isn't a figment of your imagination; it's an actual scientifically proven thing! When we've endured a long period of decision making, our ability to make good decisions fades. Our cognitive functions have simply had enough; our mental energy is depleted. At this point, we make decisions hastily or we avoid them altogether.

We're more likely to procrastinate over decisions when we're fed up with making them in the first place; with their sheer quantity, the responsibility, the lack of headspace, fear of the outcome, fearful of making a mistake, where it's an intimidating decision with big consequences, or when the topic is a source of disquiet. Perhaps, too, we just want someone to take the decision out of our hands. We're decisioned-out.

There are some decisions, though, that can't wait, can't be made by others and do require our attention sooner rather than later. But when that situation coincides with our confidence in ourselves being at an all-time low . . . that's rough.

Our mental capacity is very much like a car's fuel tank: the more you use it, the further you push it, the more depleted it gets. If you drive a car without stopping to refuel, it'll eventually splutter to a halt and do some damage to the car's internal workings. We're no different: if we use up our resources and keep pushing, we do the same.

Consequential decisions just can't be avoided but we can buy ourselves some time to restore our mental tank's fuel gauge.

Lack of Self-Awareness

So much of what we do is either on autopilot or influenced by others. We don't always pay heed to how relationships, boundaries, decisions and circumstances feel for us. Whether they truly serve us in the way we deserve for them to. And we all deserve to feel fulfilled, happy and healthy.

Self-care and self-awareness are interlinked. Self-awareness comes from self-knowledge, which is an underrated superpower. Knowing the nitty-gritty of our true selves helps us to join the dots, to spend less time dithering on trivial decisions, and to prioritise. It affords us a unique viewpoint of our world and all that's in it. We discover elements of ourselves that we didn't notice before and

'We're not the sum of our usefulness to others.'

patterns to our behaviour. When we have a rounded grasp of who we are, what's important to us, of our strengths and weaknesses, what makes us feel good and what grates on us, we develop insight into what makes us tick.

Self-awareness also allows us to change our mindset because we learn how our thoughts are leading our actions. It's understanding the 'why' in all that you do and think. It's a key part of our emotional intelligence too, giving us the vehicle with which to grow our self-confidence and providing an ongoing opportunity to check in with ourselves.

People Pleasing

There's nothing quite like rampant people pleasing to tie us up in knots. On the face of it we're being accommodating in considering the feelings and needs of others; we're expressing kindness, being selfless and willing to do anything to keep others happy. We like to feel needed, as though we matter, and so we put everyone else first and end up totally zonked out. The people who have grown accustomed to our generosity keep asking because it suits them just fine that we're so helpful, a shining asset to their lives. We give, give, give until there's nothing left to give. It's draining and stressful, and undermines our power of choice, our boundaries and our self-confidence.

Dig deeper and all that people pleasing comes from a horrible place. One where we're not comfortable in our own skins, where other people's approval holds more weight than our own, where our happiness is contingent on the happiness of others, where we don't feel we matter unless we have their validation, where we will always put others first – no matter what. Talk about a one-way ticket to Resentmentville.

We're not the sum of our usefulness to others. Oh no, we're so much more than that, and strong relationships are those that have been built on firmer foundations than how useful someone perceives us to be. It's our right to choose to carry out gestures of goodwill; they are a gift from one person to the next when we feel in control of the good deed and there are no strings attached. The difference between those gestures and people pleasing is that when we get caught up in pleasing others, we say 'yes' to their requests because we want to keep them happy; we want to prevent their anger, disappointment and rejection, to maintain the status quo. That's a 'yes' with strings attached – strings of resentment, overwhelm, guilt and pressure. Can you guess who those strings hurt? Yup, you've guessed it: us people pleasers.

Overcommitting

Modern times are hectic and loud. There's so much to think about. So much noise. It's hard to drown it out and it's difficult to feel as though we've got it under control. Data is available at our fingertips 24/7 but it means we're often available at the fingertips of others 24/7 too. We're contactable wherever we are by many means and it gets a little daunting. We've committed to more than we can possibly manage, we've shaved time from all the things we enjoy, and get by on as little sleep as possible, we push our limits and, ludicrously, we still don't feel as though we're doing enough or as though there's enough time.

We know we're overcommitted because we feel like puppets on a string. We experience an overwhelming feeling of dread at the very thought of looking at our schedules. Time blocking and colour coding mean nothing if every day, of every week, of every month, of every year is filled to the rafters. We feel as though we're time poor so we multi-task and give nothing the focus and attention it deserves. We're stressed and frazzled, and our limbs are leaden with tiredness.

We're over-committed because we're trying to cram thirty-six hours' worth of commitments into a twenty-four-hour day, every day. Our lives are nothing short of pandemonium; our responsibilities and the balls we juggle would be enough to topple us. On top of those, we have a tendency to strive for perfection in all areas of our lives, sometimes feeling as though we have something to prove, to others, and to ourselves. We find it difficult, too, to say 'no', to delegate – who would we delegate to? Our support networks are somewhat lacking.

Parenting

The reality of parenting is that it is a polarising experience; it's as fun as it is mundane, it's as rewarding as it is testing, it's as joyful as it is painful. The lessons fly at us thick and fast; we're winging it, flying by the seat of our pants.

Before we had kids, it's quite likely that we held a perfect harmonious picture in our mind's eye about the sort of parent we would be. That perfect picture of serenity didn't account for the excruciatingly steep and demanding learning curve that is parenthood. It's arguably the biggest responsibility we face and yet nothing can, nor does, prepare us for it.

There are so many things to contend with, often all at the same time; the sleep deprivation, the endless negotiating, the patience testing, the development of epic diplomacy skills, the stress, the chores, the hyper-vigilance . . . oh gosh, the list is literally endless.

We can love being parents, love our children unconditionally and still find it hard. It's the common thread between parents across the world: we're united in that 'muddling through' feeling but we don't always talk about the tough stuff. We fear judgement, scorn and criticism. This isn't limited to parenting – we don't often talk about the tough stuff we experience in life, in general. The stuff we all encounter: the rejection, the pain, the heartache and the times our heads are cobwebby, dusty sheds. Imagine how less alone we'd all feel if it were the norm to share all of that too.

As kids, we're pretty kickass at self-care. We don't hold back in expressing our needs and wants, our ups and downs.

As parents, we can learn a lot about how we react to those vocal and subtle physical cues. We protect our children's sleep time with all our might; we play the long game where energy levels are concerned too, quite often settling them down for a less taxing activity when we sense that tiredness is kicking in; we care about what they eat and drink; we consciously build in time for play; and we understand that when their needs are met, they're calmer and happier people. We bust a gut to ensure their needs are met.

It must be a bit confusing for our kids, these mixed messages we send. On the one hand, we teach them to heed their needs and bend over backwards to help them to do that, yet at the same time, we teach them that our needs are negotiable.

Being a parent doesn't have to mean the end of self-care; if anything it increases the need for it. It does take more jangling of our commitments and some clever time hacking to fit everything in. It is more difficult to keep our sense of identity as parents when we're constantly referred to as someone's mum or dad. But putting our kids first every which way doesn't teach them about boundaries, about self-respect, about respecting others' needs. We don't want our kids to model our parenting habits and turn into parents who put themselves last, over and over again. As parents, we're the leaders of our homes. Our children learn from what we say but also by what we do.

Take time to write down all the negative things
you have been told:

Now scribble over them – they're NOT your truth.
Pinky promise.

What baggage are you carrying?

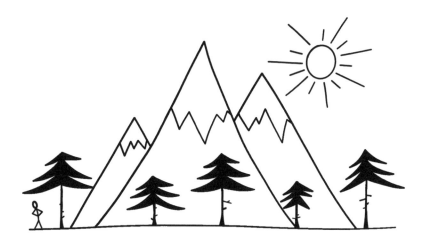

What, or who, keeps getting
in your way?

5. How to find out who we are and what we want

'We don't need fixing – we need unleashing, unpeeling, unfolding.'

The relationship we have with ourselves is *the* relationship of all our relationships, and the lynchpin. It shapes the world around us, dictates the tone of the relationships we have with others, and influences all our decisions. It's the foundation on which those other relationships are built.

When the relationship we have with ourselves is an unhealthy one, we hold the door ajar for all kinds of things to walk right on through. It's a free invitation for wonky boundaries, resentment, complications, friction, odd choices, illness, approval seeking – all manner of unsavoury things which are evidence that we might not be honouring, respecting, understanding or accepting ourselves. Our approach to this vitally important relationship isn't a particularly nourishing one; it leaves a lot to be desired, that's for sure. We unnecessarily beat ourselves up, ignore our needs, and put ourselves down. Any other relationship would struggle to survive in that toxic environment. Perhaps that *is* the undeniable truth; we *are* struggling to survive in this toxic environment. The unease, inner turmoil, conflict and brutish language aren't helping us. Not one little bit. They're keeping us small, holding us hostage to the approval of others. In shouting ourselves down, we're stunting our growth. We're creating an environment for ourselves that is scary. No wonder we're not blooming.

We burden ourselves with the 'not good enough', the 'can'ts' and the 'shoulds'; we play the same relentless, damaging and untruthful tune over and over until we can't get it out of our heads. It becomes our default outlook on who we are and what we're capable of. We don't accept ourselves, as we are, and go through life apologising for our existence; assuming that we're at fault and that those around us are faultless. We treat others like VIPs and ourselves like poo. There's discord, a mismatch, and until we address that, we're never going to master this self-care malarkey because we'll keep putting other people's needs ahead of our own. And we all know where that leads – to Sickville. Yup, nowhere we want to be heading anytime soon.

To put the 'self' into self-care, we need to design a new mixtape, dance to a new tune, adopt the teachings of our ol' friend Socrates and get to 'know thyself'. With a big dollop of self-acceptance thrown in for good measure. Only then will we be able to stop with the self-judging, the self-criticism, and see our warts for what they are – part and parcel of us but accompanied by some proper kickass strengths too. It's not up to anyone else to hand us the self-belief baton; we can only gift that to ourselves. Rejecting ourselves is futile; we are what we're born with and that has to be enough. It is enough. We are enough. As we are. It's the truest of all truths.

We don't need to be fixed – we're not broken. Lost, unsure, confused, hiding away, recovering, struggling, hurting, damaged, scarred, messy and scared, perhaps, but not broken.

It's not going to be easy to unpick and unlearn some of the really grotty habits and thought processes that we've picked up along the way. All things take time. Just as we've taken time to get to where we are, it will take time to roll up our sleeves, dig deep, question the 'why' in everything that we do, and to gain understanding about who we essentially are.

If life is a lesson, then we are the school: the facilitator of all the learning curves and the teachings, and also the chief curriculum designers.

The School of You is a place we never graduate from; we never get to leave. We're lifelong pupils. The teachers and the pupils, the bullies and the friends, are one and the same – us – we have the starring role. As for the homework – it literally never ends. Not ever. But the old adage is true: we absolutely do get out of it what we're willing to put into it. The best bit? We get to make the rules. Mwa-ha-ha!

We're malleable beings. Throughout life, we've been heavily influenced by those who brought us up: our teachers, our peers, the sum of our experiences and the media headlines. The viewpoint on who we feel we are is a borrowed one, an amalgamation of all the (often differing) perspectives, attitudes and outlooks those

'We are enough. As we are. It's the truest of all truths.'

people, and situations, have given to us. We adopt many of those viewpoints without question and they become our benchmarks, our ideals, our stance. It's like a giant game of pass the parcel where we automatically accept the views that have shaped us and don't question where they've come from. Not forgetting, of course, that those very people who influence us have inherited their views in much the same way. Our identity has been passed from pillar to post; we've picked up the quirks of generations before us and live our lives according to what they perceive as right, wrong or indifferent.

We're living someone else's version of what they believe life should be. And that probably isn't their honest version of what they believe life should be, either. They've just joined the back of the 'life should be' conga, denying themselves the space to consider if they agree or disagree.

Woah.

No wonder we feel as though we don't fit in, as though we're not enough, as though we're constantly swimming against the tide. If it feels like a chore to assert your values, they might not even be your values. If you're feeling compromised, then you most probably are being compromised – compromised by some archaic beliefs and perspectives which weren't yours to begin with. If you don't like yourself, then you probably aren't affording yourself the opportunity to be yourself – it's not you that you don't like, it's the version of you that has been shaped by others.

We don't need fixing – we need unleashing, unpeeling, unfolding.

It's a bit like drawing a line in the sand, really. Choosing to shake off those shackles, to shimmy off those labels, to earn our own respect, to stop editing who we are 'just' to fit in, to stop going against our grain, to stop following the herd.

We have more choices than we can shake a tail feather at and that's liberating and empowering, but blimey, it isn't half scary too. It's scary because it's so new and it's scary because if we're leading the way, we might go off course. We might make more mistakes, we'll be venturing into the unknown. But instead of the confinements of those inherited rules, we're now presented with options that felt invisible to us before, the limits and expectations don't weigh so heavy, possibility shimmers in the distance. Accepting ourselves as we are doesn't stunt our growth; it facilitates it.

Knowing ourselves is a revolving lesson: as we grow and change, we might need to reconnect with our evolving selves. What we once liked, we may discover we now dislike; what once nourished us might no longer help us in the same way.

Up the Self-Kindness Ante

We don't half give ourselves a hard time.

Admittedly, we live in a world that feeds into our insecurities and worries. It's easy to not feel good enough if we compare ourselves to that unlevel playing field of social feeds and the mainstream media. The highly edited photos of perfection and achievement do nothing to quieten our feelings of inadequacy; we're not as smart, not as funny, and simply not as interesting as everyone else is portrayed to be.

'Knowing ourselves is a revolving lesson.'

And we totally and utterly buy into it.

What we don't consider is for every person we feel that way about, there will be a person who feels the same way about us.

'Being kind to ourselves isn't always easy, as we feel an acute resistance to it.'

Self-kindness, then, is an act of rebellion against the 'norm'.

It's an act of rebellion against the fear that bubbles up surrounding our feelings of inadequacy, too. Fear motivates, but it's not always the best place to look for motivation. When we're motivated by fear, we're paying attention to what we don't want to happen, the things we want to avoid, the ways we might be lacking. Rather than live a life led by fear, we get to choose an alternative starting point. Kindness.

Being kind to ourselves isn't always easy, as we feel an acute resistance to it; it feels downright awkward and insincere. The about-turn from self-meanness to self-kindness is a significant one. Changing tack will always take concerted effort, patience and acceptance.

Acceptance is the magic key that opens the gateway to a less abrasive way of life. One in which we work with ourselves, and not against. We're well aware of our personality, quirks, imperfections and moods, thank you very much, but they no longer define us; they're just part and parcel of who we are. We're multifaceted and complex, and we will stumble and fall – that's a given. But when we do, we'll apply self-kindness to help us see the lesson instead of kicking ourselves when we're down. The tone we apply in our self-talk will change to one of warmth, empathy and understanding because self-kindness helps us to alleviate the stress we feel, not play into its hands. It encourages us to be sympathetic to our plights, to give ourselves the benefit of the doubt, to go easy on the berating and heavy on the love. And if love is a stretch too far, we can make a start with acceptance; acceptance that we're doing our best, have done our best, acceptance that we're different and that our differences are bloomin' marvellous assets, acceptance of our mistakes.

Become Inquisitive

As children, we question every single darn thing. Why this? Why that? Why, why, why, why, why? Our brains are absorbing new things at a rate of knots and grasping the 'why' – the mechanics of something – aids our comprehension, widens our outlook and makes us more observant.

Whilst it can be a nuisance for the adults who scrabble around trying to find answers to the squadillionth question of the day, answers that they don't always have (thank goodness for Google), sadly, somewhere along the line our inquisitive natures become a bit dampened. We start accepting things 'as is', 'falling into line', living on autopilot: a reactive life, rather than a proactive one. It means we probably do things and think things with no idea as to their basis, the 'why'. This is also when we feel powerless, as though so much of what happens is out of our control.

Scientific discoveries, innovation, creativity and advances in technology are all born from a curious mind. It's a good habit for us to reintroduce into our daily lives, this curiosity factor (and no, it did not kill the cat). Challenging our assumptions, others' assumptions, the stories we tell ourselves, the way the world around us works and indeed, the world at large. Questions are our friends: they illuminate answers, uncover options available to us, encourage us to try new things, give us an understanding of what our motivators are, make room for differing perspectives, move us out of stagnation and complacency, challenge stereotypes, facilitate our growth, and force us to be mindful.

With all the rules/limits/expectations/assumptions we absorb from the people around us, it's more important than ever to keep questioning the 'why' and to keep revisiting that question, because the 'why' may well alter with time. Doing so gives us the chance to keep realigning our actions with who we are, who we want to be, and what we want to do.

Use Envy as a Signpost

Our lives, should we choose for them to be, are sliced and diced across social media. We know more about the comings and goings of our peers now than we ever did before. We've got a front-row ticket to the Humblebrag show and that's not all it's cracked up to be. Especially for those of us who err towards not feeling 'enough' in the first place.

Social media is rife with validation-seeking posts and is a hotbed of comparisonitis, but the comparison isn't always a fair one. We're not armed with all the information needed to make a fair comparison – we end up comparing where we are, in all its realness and unpolished-ness, with a microsecond snapshot of someone's best bits. We'll see the achievement, but not the pain of the journey to get there; the rejection, the late nights, the anguish, the balancing, the growth. We'll see a group shot where everyone is smiling at the camera with their cheesy grins and twinkly eyes, but we don't see the spats, the resentment, the unspoken angst, the heartache. We see photos of beautiful bonnie babies but we don't see the sleepless nights, the anguish of whether to return to work, the self-doubt, the anxiety, the trepidation. We see a selfie and feel inadequate, but we don't see the self-esteem issues, the uncertainty, the insecurity and the filters behind it.

We take these images at face value and we make snap judgements based on those snapshots of a micro moment in time, but we don't consider that the grass isn't always greener. We don't read between the lines, consider that our perspective might be a bit squiffy, or consider what's not being said. The snapshot becomes the benchmark with which we compare ourselves and it can be a rough ride. The bar feels as though it's been set high and once again, we don't match up.

Rather than beat ourselves up (remember, we're practising self-kindness), rather than encasing those envious feelings in shame, we can explore them, let them guide us. Those pangs of envy we feel can be indicative of where we want to go, who we want to be and what we'd like to achieve. Envy is an incredible tool that's at our disposal; it highlights our dreams, our needs, the possibilities and opportunities we might not have considered, and it reminds us of our desires. It can present you with a redirection signal, too; perhaps there is an alternative way to work towards your dreams and aspirations.

Whatever we feel is what we feel. No emotions are wrong or bad. It's how we interpret the messages they give us that matters, and then, what we choose to do with that information.

Start a Journal

Remember those diaries we kept as teenagers? The ones covered in doodles and stickers? The notebooks that became laden with our secrets, our hopes and our angst as we navigated the somewhat turbulent, confusing, frightening, ever-changing and steep learning curve that is adolescence. The books that we stored under our mattresses and floorboards because the very worst thing that could happen would be for someone to discover our deepest, darkest secrets and reveal them to all and sundry, leading to social pariah status.

Why did we ever stop that? The outpouring of our emotions, the reflection, the honesty, the self-expression, the brain-dumping, the slower pace of life for a micro moment, and the space to just be?

Journaling isn't just an excuse to buy some snazzy new stationery (as if we ever need an excuse for that!). It's an act of self-care, a powerful tool which allows us the space to get to grips with what's going on for us, in real time.

When we give ourselves the quiet space to write, whether that be letting the words flow or in response to some journal prompts, whether it be throughout the

'the reflection, the honesty, the self-expression, the brain-dumping, the slower pace of life for a micro moment, and the space to just be'

day, in the morning or the evening, we hush the dialogue of the outside world and tune into our internal dialogue. We increase its volume and that's super helpful because it gives us the chance to discover how we truly feel about things, to dial in on patterns of thinking and behaviour, to work through our layers and see what comes up. Journaling helps us to identify triggers, those times our boundaries were compromised, the times we asserted our boundaries, areas of our lives we need more support with, unexpected happy moments, solutions to problems, our 'wins', our unmet needs, dreams we'd forgotten about: it helps us to join the dots.

When we call on our memories to reflect on a period of time, it's often polarised recall; we remember the very best bits and the very worst bits. When we capture our thoughts and feelings on a regular basis, we also capture the middle ground and that can be illuminating in so many ways. Seeing our emotions, the sources of stress, the feelings, the accomplishments, the celebrations, the troubles and the strife, in black and white, validates them and helps us to view them objectively.

There is no right or wrong way to journal – only *your* way – you get to decide. It's a chance to unplug, regroup, unwind. Some much needed 'me time'. There's no need to stumble over spelling, punctuation and grammar, either; this precious time is all about shaking off the confines of life, to partake in self-exploration and expression.

Listen to How You Feel

Now then, we often write this sort of stuff off as a bit 'woo-woo', as we prefer concrete evidence that makes logical sense. But as people, we just don't make sense; we're complex creatures. We have instincts, hunches and hackles that are wiser than we give them credit for. We experience physical sensations in reaction to situations: increased heart rate, tension, sweaty palms, altered breathing and a knot in our stomachs. We acknowledge those sensations because they're downright uncomfortable and we try to rationalise them but we don't always listen to what they're telling us.

We've already established that there are times when we feel torn, conflicted or pulled in different directions. In addition to the societal 'shoulds' and 'oughts' that sway us, our brains operate in such a way that the two sides don't always agree. You see, one half of our brain operates on an analytical level, taking into consideration all the conscious experiences and data to hand, in a slow, measured way. The second half of our brain operates in a flash of light, delving into our subconscious filing cabinets, and doesn't always come up with answers that make rational sense. Both sides serve us differently depending on the circumstances and neither side is foolproof; we only know what we know and we can weigh up decisions only with this knowledge.

Self-care demands that we're in tune with how we feel and how we want to feel. At times, a short-term decision we need to make will conflict with the long game. We're trying to get those in sync – not always possible, but a good stance to begin with.

We all know how our feelings can change depending on circumstances; how we feel after spending time with people who energise us and how we feel after spending time with people who drain us, how we feel when we've agreed to do something that wonkifies our boundaries and instantly a ball of dread forms in our stomachs, the butterflies of excitement, the butterflies of nerves, those ignored dreams that gnaw away at us, the times when we've blushed uncontrollably, the times we've felt restored, comforted and nourished.

In ignoring how we feel about things – what feels right and what doesn't feel right – we're ignoring a way of helping us decide what self-care is, and isn't, for us as individuals; ignoring a wise evolutionary tool which helps us to make decisions based on what we instinctively know to be right for us.

Start a Scrapbook

'Who am I?' is arguably one of the toughest questions to answer because we don't always know. It's a humungous question that often prompts more questions than it does answers. Sadly, we may have never known the answer; we may have experienced situations that have put our identity into question or found ourselves at rock bottom due to trauma and/or illness. We may have become so used to living to please others that we don't know how else to be. Society tries to squish us all into labelled boxes, boxes that we simply don't fit into, nor do we want to.

Our sense of self, the quest to understand who we are, is an inherent need. We're driven by a thirst to understand our core identities, even if we don't realise it. Our sense of identity is the overarching understanding we have of ourselves: our strengths, weaknesses, likes, dislikes, values, hobbies, etc. It's important because it grounds us, acts as our internal compass and helps us to make decisions. When we're unsure of who we

'Starting a scrapbook of 'you' is a visual way of piecing your identity together.'

fundamentally are, we feel adrift, disorientated and unsettled. It feels as though we're wearing a mask and we're vulnerable to being controlled by external factors, which affects how we see ourselves and, in turn, our sense of wellbeing.

Who we are also changes; we're not now who we were five, ten, twenty years ago. We evolve, we change, and we take on new roles.

Starting a scrapbook of 'you' is a visual way of piecing your identity together. One idea is to find pictures/photos/visual representations of your answers to questions such as: 'What's important to me?', 'Who do I enjoy spending time with, and why?', 'What are my favourite things?', 'What comforts me?', 'Where would I like to travel/explore?', 'What does my ideal day look like?', 'What did I want to be when I was younger?', 'What are my favourite songs?', 'What hobbies do I enjoy?', 'What is holding me back?', 'What new things would I like to try?' and 'What colours/flowers/foods am I drawn to?' The list of possible questions is endless. What's so useful about this method of self-discovery is that the questions seem relatively simple in isolation, but, combined, they make up the answers to the big question – who am I?

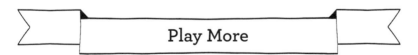

Play More

Where children are concerned, play is where it's at and it's the kids who don't play that we worry about. Play is fun but also a highly encouraged gateway to learning. Not only is it good for our cognitive skills but also our interactions with others, our emotional wellbeing, our problem-solving skills and our imagination.

Let's face it, adulting isn't at all what it's cracked up to be. We're full to the brim with responsibility, we've bought into the social status of busyness, devalued anything that we enjoy, are constantly constrained by an overflowing to-do list, and we're bored of being bored, and of being so darn serious. At some point, we chose work over play, monotony over exploration, tasks over fun, boredom over pleasure.

We blame time, that there's not enough of it. It's the lie we spin ourselves but we find time for everything else and everyone else: work, family, friends, chores, watching television, numerous social media check-ins, emergencies. The truth is that to prioritise fun makes us feel guilty, frivolous and indulgent. Sometimes, it's so far removed from what we feel, we just can't buy into it. It's been so long since we did things just for the joy and pleasure of them that we lose sight of its benefits. And make no bones about it; we're never too old to play and we're never too old to reap its benefits. With stress-related illnesses on the increase at an alarming intensity, we can't really afford *not* to make time for stress-busting play any more – there's too much at stake.

We don't forget how to play; we just get out of the habit of it. It's not linked to a specific outcome – it's unstructured and unproductive, and takes us away from our responsibilities. The reasons we give ourselves for not doing it are exactly the counter-arguments *for* play.

Find an image,
or draw an image
which represents
how you feel
right now

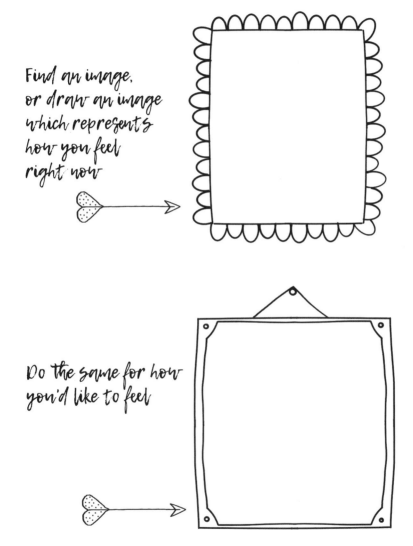

Do the same for how
you'd like to feel

[your name here]

_____'s favourite things

Use the boxes below to describe yourself in 10 positive words

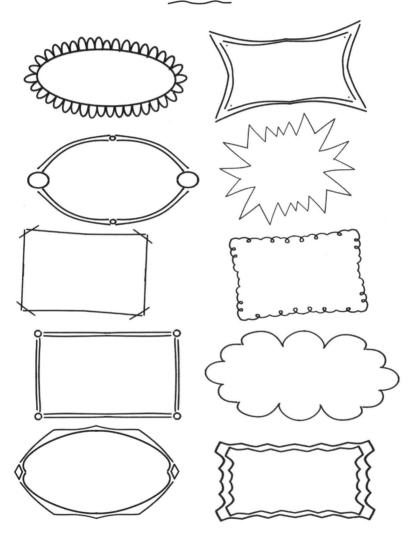

6. We don't have to go 'all-in': the power of the micro

'We're going to take back our power, in teeny tiny steps.'

Arriving at the point where we agree that self-care is beneficial is just the start. It's a fantastic start but it's figuring out how to make it a sustained and long-term part of our lives where the difficulty lies.

The thought of doing something new can be nothing short of gigantic in our mind's eye. We look at whatever 'it' is as it looms over us and we either go 'all-in', and find it difficult to maintain the changes required, or we feel paralysed by it. Not knowing where to begin, quite often we don't begin. We don't make a start and it becomes another thing we've procrastinated on, another dent to our self-esteem. Even when that 'thing' might well be something we've identified as being important to us – something that might help us to feel more confident, joyful, inspired, nourished, strong, etc. – its importance doesn't belie the fact it feels scary to venture down an unbeaten path.

'The unknown is a common fear for many.'

Our mind can work for and against us. Acknowledging that we want to change and going about it are two very different things. We feel an insurmountable resistance.

This is partly down to fear: fear of the unknown, fear of failure and fear that we're not enough. We all have a fear radar which lurks inside us, scanning for threats and dangers. Once it has fixed its sights on a threat, it sends warning messages to the rest of our body. Fear is unequivocally useful at times; when our lives really are at risk. We wouldn't be without it then, but the trouble with our fear radar is that it has been known to have performance issues – it can be a little dodgy, a tad unreliable. This fear radar detects danger based on imaginary scenarios of how something might play out. It computes all possible scenarios and prepares us for what 'might' lie ahead. That's right; our body will react to a perceived unfavourable outcome in exactly the same way it would react to a sabre-toothed tiger on the prowl nearby. The radar initiates a set of physiological processes which prime us for fight or flight. We may experience butterflies in our stomachs, our hackles rise, adrenaline courses through our veins, we become hyper-alert and hyper-vigilant.

The unknown is a common fear for many of us as it calls for us to step outside our comfort zones where we, you know, feel comfortable. It calls for us to do something different from what we've done before with no guarantees of what the outcome will be. Fear steps in and magnifies the potential negative outcomes. It predicts, and convincingly argues against, the proposed future changes based on some pretty shoddy anecdotal evidence. Fear's evolutionary aim is to keep us safe, which incidentally can also keep us small, hold us prisoner and shackle us to our insecurities. A life with fear at the helm ain't a very happy one.

Fear puts a strain on us. All we're trying to do is to write our own stories, carve out a better life for ourselves, choose which paths we'd like to take. But fear throws a spanner in the works and becomes a feisty opponent.

The good news is that fear needn't remain in control; we can shove it out of the way, build up resilience to it and take steps to overcome its power.

To loosen fear's grip on us and to expand our comfort zones, we need to initiate 'courage' mode. Yup, we're going to have to roll up our sleeves and prepare to change how this story pans out. We're going to take back our power, in teeny tiny steps. Steps and moments so minuscule that, alone, they barely register. Being courageous sounds ginormous, but all it really takes is micro acts and micro moments of bravery. Just as it takes micro acts and micro moments of resisting the story that fear tells us for us to become resilient to it. The more of those micro acts and micro moments we accumulate, the easier it becomes to flex and adapt, we feel increasingly stronger and more confident, we get more comfortable with the uncomfortable and, before we know it, we've cemented some new habits. Win, win.

And fret not, fear, we're not going to ignore you, you don't have to shout louder to be heard. We hear you all right, but we can also see you *'Get more comfortable* for what you are. We see your flaws *with the uncomfortable.'* and we'll offer a nod of recognition.

But we're also going to square up to you and then show you who's boss.

It *is* an inner battle; to some intents and purposes, we are at war with ourselves. It's also no mean feat. It draws on our mental faculties but in taking the smallest steps possible, we'll also be allowing plenty of time for our energy levels to build back up.

We're all well versed in knowing which behaviours are most likely to produce positive results. The finicky bit is where our current behaviours feel like light years away from what we would like our behaviours to be. And don't think for one minute that our brains will make it easy for us either; our brains prefer our existing habits, to stick with what they know, and aren't supportive of our goals. They're designed to help us take the easy way out, the path of least resistance, and when we want to make changes, we're not just using up more mental resources; we're also fighting against some formidable neural pathways. And so we're going to have to hack that automation in a sustained, realistic and relatively simple way.

We're going to play the long game.

And that's not as easy as it sounds.

We tend to rush progress – it's that instant gratification thing where we know what we want and we want it now, without delay. Right now. Right this second. Once we've made up our minds about something, we don't want to have to wait. We don't have to wait for much these days: we can instant-message our friends, order items online for same-day delivery, and be in a different country within hours. The problem with instant gratification is that in seeking the short-term pleasure of it, we might be foregoing long-term happiness. The opposite is true, too;

long-term pleasure means we sometimes have to be willing to forego the short-term happiness.

Sounds pretty darn dissatisfying, right?

Imagine, if you will, the sea. There's no denying it's a powerful beast but it's not by sheer force and power that it erodes a cliff face. Nope, the damage is done by the incessant waves over a long period of time, chipping away at the cliff one by one. Wave by wave. Slowly but surely.

Instant gratification is short-sighted. It's an inability to see long term and to muster the patience to see our plans play out. Going 'all-in' can sometimes lead to us setting unrealistic goals, comparable to climbing Mount Everest with no prior preparation or training. When we bite off more than we can chew, we unwittingly and unnecessarily set ourselves up for failure and it hurts. Our failures can teach us a fair bit, but we rarely give them much airtime and with all the good will in the world, if failure becomes a habit we don't learn something from then that's destructive. Unheeded failure can be a menace. If we continue to make the same mistakes over and over, without looking for lessons and the messages they contain, our self-confidence slowly erodes over time. We become unwilling to try new things; failure seems like a pre-determined outcome. And it's absolutely not a pre-determined outcome. Nothing is – we all screw up but we wouldn't be able to walk if, as babies, we hadn't stumbled, flexed, and kept trying. Failure doesn't have to equal defeat; it doesn't have to be the end of the road. Understanding why we failed and reflecting on what we might

'Long-term pleasure means we sometimes have to be willing to forego the short-term happiness.'

have done differently helps us to connect the dots, to form a new roadmap. It gives us data that makes our second, third, fourth, hundredth attempts more likely to succeed.

'Micro actions require minimal effort, motivation, energy and ability.'

Implementing a new habit, even one as beneficial and metamorphic as making time for self-care, doesn't happen overnight. Habits are formed by repeated actions and when those planned actions are too big, too disruptive, it can feel a little chaotic. Our knee-jerk reaction is to return to the 'norm', back to what we know and what we're used to. Back to square one.

When we repeatedly find ourselves back at square one, our motivation starts to deplete and our willpower starts to waver. It takes mental energy to pick ourselves up time and time again, to dust off and start again. It's the starting that is so exhausting.

That's why micro actions and micro moments make complete and utter sense. They are almost always realistic – that's the beauty of them. They don't require a huge overhaul but as their momentum builds, they have the potential to bring about massively positive changes. Micro actions require minimal effort, motivation, energy and ability. The smaller the action, the more achievable it feels and the easier it is to build into our everyday lives. There's no need to rifle through our already-crammed schedules to find chunks of time to change; we can always find time for a micro moment of self-care. And if we're already frazzled, there are even micro actions we can take from the comfort of our own bed!

Change can be uncomfortable but micro actions grant us the grace to change in increments. There's no need to limber up; you won't be asking a lot of yourself. You won't need to leap, jump, run or hurdle.

We're talking about taking tentative steps into the unknown, finding our bearings and then crawling forward rather than taking a big ungainly gallop. We're in many ways slowing down progress but also increasing our chances of long-term success, making bigger strides than it feels as though we are.

To identify what micro action or micro moment to take, we need to commit to a goal, a dream, or a desired feeling. That's the outcome, the result we'd like to end up at. Next, we need to brainstorm the teeniest steps we might take to get there and list these somewhere we can refer back to. This is called reverse engineering – we're taking the end product and breaking it down until we have a series of tiny and manageable steps to help us to get there.

The actions and moments don't take a lot of time or energy. They slot easily into our daily schedule. They don't add more pressure. If we miss a micro action or micro moment, it's not a big deal – it's easy to get back on the wagon. They're manageable slices of time which keep us focused on our chosen outcome in amongst the loudness that is life. As we layer the micro actions and micro moments, we notice ever-so-subtle shifts in our lives; we experience more 'wins'. Our confidence builds, as does the momentum and impact.

In terms of building self-care into our daily lives, this is a strategy that is achievable, captivating, rewarding and encouraging. The accumulation of daily pockets of intentional action and moments helps us to push through the fear and resistance we feel.

There are pockets of 'dead' time in all of our daily lives.

Pockets of time when we're commuting, waiting for an appointment, on hold or lurking on Facebook, which we can use to our advantage and hijack for some micro moments of self-care.

Because that's the basis of self-care: not that it adds to the stresses and strains of the day, but that it reduces them. And pockets of time afford us the opportunity to pause, to reflect and to take stock.

It's surprising what can be achieved in a micro moment, or in a series of micro moments, and whilst what counts as self-care will be different for each and every one of us, these are some things we can do which totally fall under the self-care umbrella, which could benefit us all.

Inbox Clearout

Even with the best intentions in the world, our inboxes are often overflowing: the emails we need to reply to, the emails we don't remember subscribing to, and the emails we need to save for another day. We've got emails coming out of our ears.

They're often disruptive, interrupting whatever it is that we're focusing on with their incessant alerts and making us hop to the beat of our smartphone notifications, rather than our surroundings.

Self-care calls for us to take back control of what we do, and when we do it, and email makes that tricky. To take back some control over email, there are a few things we can do:

'Pockets of time afford us the opportunity to pause, to reflect and to take stock.'

- Remove the capacity to send/receive emails from our

smartphones, or at the very least, silence the notifications we receive so that we consciously choose when to check in.

- Keep the browser or the email application closed when working on our desktop and check in at set periods throughout the day.
- Use a service like unroll.me to mass-unsubscribe from mailing lists (often ones we don't remember signing up for).
- Set up email folders for historic emails that are clogging up our inbox so that we can lay our hands on the emails we're after easily.

Drink Some Water

Our body is made up of two-thirds water – it's important to keep those levels boosted so that we function at our optimum: our temperature is regulated, vitamins, minerals and oxygen are moved around where needed, etc. By the time we're experiencing dehydration-related headaches, our water levels have dipped and need to be topped up. Being dehydrated, even ever so slightly, affects our bodily functions, our mood, our productivity and our brainpower.

It can be difficult to remember to drink regularly throughout the day and the noise of life often masks some of the body's cues that it needs more fluid. One way we can get our smartphones to work for us, instead of against us, is to install an app which will remind us to have a drink and tally up what we've had to drink throughout the day.

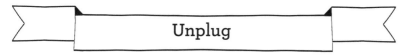

Unplug

The arm bone is connected to the hand bone. The hand bone's connected to the finger bone. The finger bone's connected to the smartphone. All day long. Well, perhaps not all day, but a great big chunk of it. We're replying, liking, scrolling, lurking and checking in a staggering seventy six times a day on average.

The blue light that our phones emit has been linked to insomnia – it's believed that the blue light suppresses the production of melatonin, which is a hormone our body produces to induce sleep. Disrupted and poor-quality sleep can be caused by late-night scrolling.

Being a slave to our electronic devices is no fun at all. It makes sense to unplug before bedtime, but also at other times throughout the day. Doing so allows us space and silence, time slows down, we notice more around us, connect better with those who are in the room, connect better with ourselves and feel less on edge.

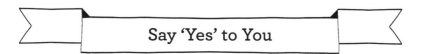

Say 'Yes' to You

The demands on our time are fast and furious. We could literally fill each day several times over. In fact, that's just what we do. We fill our time with the demands of others and an abundance of responsibilities. Before we know it, time has flown by in the blink of an eye. We can't rewind time, we can't magic up more time but we can get smart about how we use it and how it works for us.

We've already considered the times we say 'yes' to others when we feel pressured to, when we feel as though we ought to, or out of guilt, but we've not yet touched on the times we say 'no' to the things that light us up. The times we say 'no' to ourselves, compromising our health, our dreams, and the relationships that matter to us.

When we put ourselves last all the darn time, we're showing others that's our place. But it's not; we're as important as the next person and deserve opportunities to do the things that matter to us. It's perfectly acceptable to decline a request to work late because we want to spend time with our friends and family. It's perfectly reasonable not to answer the telephone if we're in the middle of a good book. It's fair to ask people not to turn up at our homes unannounced. It's commendable when we protect the time we've set aside to work towards our dreams.

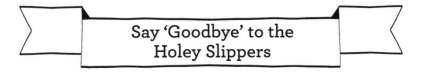

Say 'Goodbye' to the Holey Slippers

When we feel worthless, we feel unworthy of anyone's time and attention, we feel unworthy of friendship, we feel unworthy of help and we feel unworthy of 'nice things'.

The fraying and greying underwear, the slippers which have more holes than a cheese grater, the beautiful china that we save for the special occasions. We make do.

But we don't have to.

We deserve the slippers that keep our feet warm, we deserve underwear that makes us feel swit swoo and we deserve to treat every day as though it is a special occasion, because we're special. When we replace the tatty items one by one, we're challenging some ingrained thoughts. Our actions are speaking louder than our words. We're telling ourselves we are worthy, because we are. We always are.

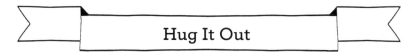

Hug It Out

Ah, the humble hug! We've been hugging our way through life since we were nippers. We hug people, we hug pets, we hug blankets and we hug our teddy bears.

Hugs are magic; they comfort, they calm and they reassure. When we hug someone we care about, the benefits of hugging increase. The longer the hug, the better. A big squeeze is nothing short of medicinal; a twenty-second hug will release a hormone called oxytocin (the love hormone). Oxytocin is credited with decreasing our heart rate, lowering our blood pressure, giving relief from pain, lowering the production of cortisol (the stress hormone), stimulating the production of dopamine (the pleasure hormone) and increasing our sense of belonging.

Arms at the ready . . . SQUISH!

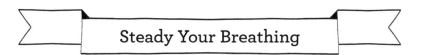

Steady Your Breathing

We don't always notice this, but when we're stressed, nervous and anxious, our breathing changes. It speeds up and we don't breathe as deeply as we did when we were feeling calmer.

The instant we turn our focus to our breath, we switch into mindfulness mode – we're transported into the present moment and it's difficult to think of anything else if we're truly focusing on the breath as we inhale and exhale. That's why so many guided meditations start with this exercise; it pulls our attention to the 'now' and when we're fully in the 'now' it's harder to be stressed, nervous and anxious about something outside that.

We all feel stressed occasionally and can plan ahead by installing apps, such as Breathe2Relax (free), on our phone, ready to help us when we need them. A really simple exercise we can do without an app is to breathe in through the nose to the count of five and then to breathe out through the mouth to the count of five. Repeat until you feel your heart rate return to normal.

Keep Up the Boring Self-Care Stuff

The boring, yet vital, self-care stuff can lurk in our brains, relying on memory alone. The trouble with our memories is that the days merge into one and there's so much already stored in there to be completed. It's easy to get caught up in life and to forget the important stuff. We're talking about appointments, prescriptions, taking your medication, getting enough sleep, paying bills and filling out forms.

Setting up reminders for these things on our smartphones lets our brains off the hook. It can free up headspace and automate the remembering bit of the self-care process. We don't have to worry that we've forgotten to do X, Y and Z because the reminders have got our backs and will let us know what we need to do, and when, in due course. Once again, letting our smartphones work for us.

Create a Bedtime Routine

Sleep is a non-negotiable act of self-care, yet we seem to be making less and less time for it.

A lack of sleep has far-reaching consequences; it undermines our wellbeing and affects our cognitive functions in such a way that sleep deprivation has been used as a means of torture throughout history. We're putting ourselves at risk – emotionally, mentally and physically – when we forego sleep.

This period of rest and recovery is a thing of beauty; it facilitates learning and memory, boosts our immunity, reduces stress, prevents accidents, manages our appetite, decreases our risk of disease and keeps us happy.

In creating a bedtime routine, we can protect this portion of our day, increase the effectiveness of our sleep and increase our chances of waking up feeling refreshed and raring to go. Because let's face it, that's not the current norm for us.

A bedtime routine might start throughout the day; we might build in some rest breaks, avoid caffeine after 2 p.m., limit sugar, limit screen time after 8 p.m., tweak our sleep environment so it's comfortable, and review what time we might need to turn in in order to get the recommended seven to nine hours of sleep. Other things we might consider are: going to bed and getting up at the same time every day, beginning to wind down thirty minutes before bed, turning our phones off and charging them in a different room overnight, drinking some hot milk, reading, listening to soothing music, journaling, or having a warm bath or shower.

Make a Playlist

Music brings us together, evokes memories, resonates, soothes, motivates, reassures and comforts. It can also decrease our blood pressure, boost mental wellbeing, elevate our mood, increase alertness, reduce anxiety, decrease stress and help us to exercise with more gusto.

Musical tastes vary from person to person; we react in different ways to different melodies and lyrics. There are different tunes that make up the soundtracks to our lives; there will be songs that evoke painful memories, those that resonate with the tough stuff we've been through, those that make us smile, those that make us want to shimmy underneath a sparkly disco ball, those that make us feel happy, those that offer us a reprieve from the day-to-day drivel, and those that boost our confidence.

As with all self-care activities, the key is in the planning, which might affect the songs on our playlist and whether we compile more than one. For instance, we could put together a playlist for a rainy day, for a sucky day, for the times we need to be energised, for the times we need a steady stream of confidence-boosting tracks, perhaps to help unleash some feistiness, to provide hope, for when we're angry, for when we're sad, for romance, for friendship, for giggles.

Shake It Like a Polaroid Picture

Planning exercise into an already chock-a-block schedule can feel impossible. It can also be eye roll inducing to even suggest exercise when we feel so darn depleted as it is. We're already wiped out, thanks. But exercise doesn't have to be a solid hour in a sweaty gym to still be effective; exercise can be rejuvenating, help with circulation, aid our immune system, help us to decompress, and calm us. And we can feel the benefits from pockets of time here and there – it doesn't have to be in one big block that we dread.

Finding a way that works for us is key, whether that's a fifteen-minute caper around the block at lunch-time or a longer gallivant in the hills, shaking it like a polaroid picture to our favourite cheesy tunes, doing star-jump windmill-arms cycling-legs circuits, jumping on a trampoline or space-hopper, doing YouTube yoga, following a Davina DVD, surfing . . . The only important aspects are that it's enjoyable and that we'll do it.

Let's not be afraid to do it our way.

'Exercise doesn't have to be a solid hour in a sweaty gym to still be effective.'

We all have fears, use the signposts to name yours

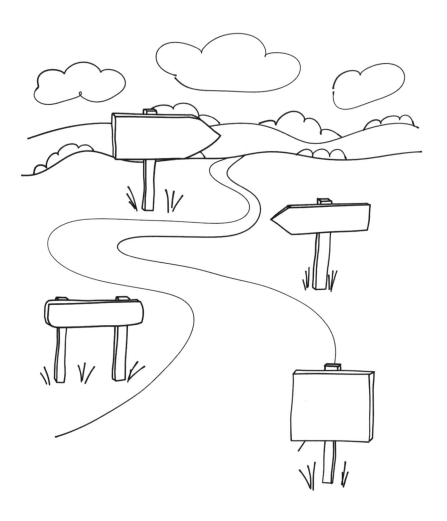

Name your acts of bravery

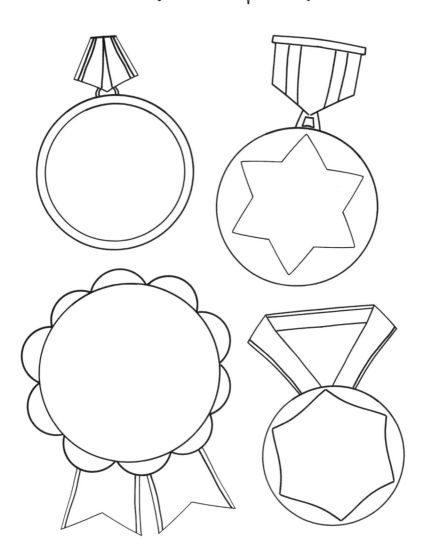

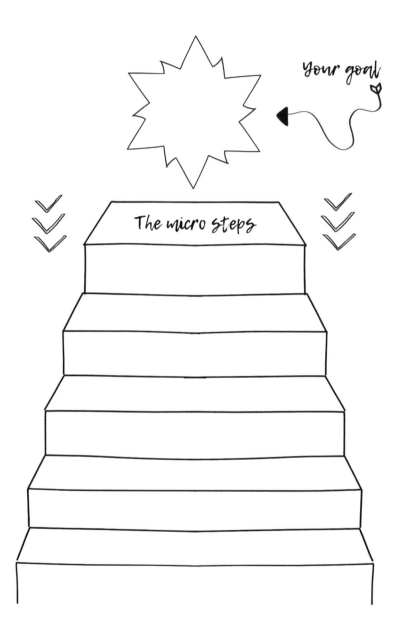

7. Prioritising and planning self-care into our already busy lives

'We sideline our needs until "some" day, and "some" day never arrives.'

There's a saying that goes something like this: 'Prior planning prevents p*ss-poor performance'. But we're going to reframe it (because we can) to say: 'Prior planning prevents poor health and wonky boundaries' (because it does). When we drop the self-care ball (because we will) that's not poor performance, it's life. It's going to happen, of that there is no doubt, but we're going to look at how to plan for the ball to stay up in the air for as long as possible. And we're not going to beat ourselves up for dropping the self-care ball, either; we're just going to pick it right back up again and again and again and again.

This is arguably the most important chapter of this book because it's the one where the difference is truly made. It's also the chapter that can feel a little intimidating because the baton is well and truly in our hands now. We have a renewed understanding of self-care, and of ourselves. It's what we do with this precious information which counts.

It's one thing understanding why we want to change things, wanting desperately to do so, and quite another to keep that fire in our bellies stoked so that we take the action needed to change. After all, life is just a series of micro decisions and micro moments and if we can be mindful and self-aware about those, we can make some pretty cool changes. One teeny tiny step at a time.

Sounds easy-ish, doesn't it?!

But it's not.

Why?

Life trips us up, we trip ourselves up, other people trip us up, our brain works against us. Old habits creep back in. It's tiring going against the grain to change and cement new habits; it takes self-discipline, motivation and willpower, and those aren't in never-ending supply.

And the thing about self-care is that the more we do it, the more we feel its transformative magic, and the more we're going to want to do it, to make other changes – and so that friction of going against the grain doesn't go away; we just learn to get comfy with it.

To give ourselves the best possible chance of change, we need to put our planning hats on.

Cue the eye roll.

It's true, planning sounds unsexy, restrictive, boring and like bloody hard work. And we've had enough of the boring and hard work, thank you very much!

But we plan for every other area of our lives: work, school, birthdays, holidays, weddings, children, retirement, etc. Why wouldn't we have a plan that enables us to function at our best? A plan that puts us firmly back in the driving seat and one that anchors us when it feels as though the world is conspiring against our health and our goals. A plan that encapsulates and prioritises our needs and wants, highlights what we want to say 'yes' to and what we want to say 'no' to, but also affords the opportunity to rewrite our future based on how the past has shaped our present.

Unfortunately, self-care doesn't materialise as happenstance – it only works if we are intentional about it.

But we don't have time for this!

No, it certainly doesn't feel like it. We're overwhelmed by all the chores, stuff, people, noise that already scream for our attention. Self-care, at this point, feels like pie in the sky. Unachievable and unattainable.

Let's start by seeing if we can loosen up some time and headspace.

Renegotiate Smartphone Time

One of the greatest time-sucker-uppers today is social media. It's undoubtedly a fantastic tool in many ways but its very nature means than we often underestimate the time we spend on it. We allegedly check our phones as often as seventy-six times a day and we can feel quite defensive about that too. We're not looking to cut it out completely, not at all; we're looking to see what time we can shave off it. If we could reduce that to, say, twenty-five times, then we've already found a cheeky pocket of time for some self-care shenanigans. Remember, it's those micro pockets of time that we're reaching for.

There are apps we can install which will give us data about how much time we're spending on our smartphones – AntiSocial and Moment are two fantastic apps which help with this. Remember, the aim of this data isn't to make us feel ashamed or guilty; there is no right or wrong amount of time to spend on social media, there's only what works for us as individuals. For some of us it's the only interaction we have with others, our only window into the outside world; we might need to use it for work, to give and receive support, to keep up with the news, to learn, to check in with accountability groups. This is not another stick with which to beat ourselves; it's just to give us an accurate estimate of where our time might be going so that we can renegotiate that time, if we *want* to. If going on social media is an act of self-care in that it helps us to feel good, nourished, comforted and energised, then we might as well skip this step completely – we've got this base covered.

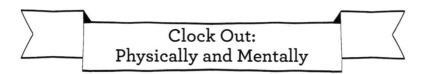

Clock Out:
Physically and Mentally

Another common time-dissolving area is the blurred line between work time and personal space. 'Work–life balance' is a term that's bandied about and can lead us to feel as though we've failed before we've even begun. There is just no such steady thing as balance – the conditions don't all meet up in a perfect spot; they're fluid. There isn't an emotional or mental door we can close once we've clocked off from work, just as we don't forget about our families whilst we're at work. These parts of our lives mesh and blend but more so when we love our jobs, work from home, work flexitime or feel pressure to make ourselves available 24/7.

In isolation, this isn't a big deal; it's barely noticeable. But our hours of work are creeping into our non-work time, on a regular basis. They're expanding and encroaching on time that's designed to be downtime, the time when we can focus on non-work things and have some fun. There isn't always a clear distinction between where work ends and our personal time begins.

Straighten Those Wonky Boundaries

When we feel as though the differing elements and people in our lives all merge into one, then it's quite likely down to wonky boundaries; ours and other people's.

Whether we realise it or not, we all have boundaries; the physical, emotional and mental lines that dictate to ourselves, and to those around us, what we will and will not allow or tolerate. They influence how we might behave and how we expect others to treat us and behave around us. They're powerful things, these boundaries – they protect us and set the tone for all relationships, the personal ones and the work ones, the healthy and not-so-healthy ones.

We experience boundaries every day, in all we do. For example,

'It's our right, and responsibility, to decide what our limits are and then to communicate and assert those boundaries.'

boundaries tell us not to walk up to a stranger and help ourselves to a lick of their ice cream, nor walk into a stranger's house, uninvited, and run ourselves a bath. We also see examples of boundaries being pushed; an employer who regularly expects a response outside contracted work hours, who sets unrealistic targets and timeframes. We wouldn't ordinarily walk up to a stranger and touch their stomach, yet some people feel it's perfectly acceptable to walk up to a pregnant lady and do just that (it's not acceptable, not without permission).

It's our right, and responsibility, to decide what our limits are and then to communicate and assert those boundaries. We may experience resistance from others when we assert our boundaries, or we might feel resistance when other people assert theirs. They work both ways; we must respect the boundaries of others as much as they must respect ours.

We know when our boundaries have been compromised because we feel as though we're in a real-life pinball machine, bouncing this way, that way, forwards and backwards, swayed by other people's wants, needs and demands of us. We feel taken advantage of, manipulated, as though we've got 'mug' written on our foreheads. We feel disrespected and experience anger, confusion, frustration and annoyance.

Healthy boundaries are the difference between saying 'yes' because we feel we ought to (it's that Law of Should, again) and saying 'no' because we mean 'no'. If we don't know what our boundaries are, what we will and won't tolerate, we can't expect others to know what they might be, either. We need to get clear on what matters to us, what we will and won't accept.

As much as boundaries protect, they can also isolate. They can be wonky, but they can be restrictive and claustrophobic. We know when our boundaries are of the fortress type too because we feel misunderstood, lonely, disconnected and isolated from others. The walls we've built to protect us, to keep others at arm's length, can also feel like the walls of a prison.

Boundaries allow us to maintain our individuality, to communicate our needs clearly, to change our minds, and to live in alignment with our identity. They allow us the space we need to grow, to recharge, and to take care of our needs. They provide a blueprint that helps us to plan in plentiful time for the things that matter to us.

Give Multi-Tasking the Heave-Ho

We talk about multi-tasking as though it's an art to be mastered and when we feel we've got it sussed, we don't half feel proud of ourselves.

It seems to be the golden ticket to a promised land of empty inboxes and completed to-do lists where we can kick back and relax, basking in our productivity skills.

There's bad news, folks: there's no such thing as multi-tasking. *Wh-wh-what?!*

Scientists have discovered that we can never truly do more than one thing at a time; our brains just can't handle it. Instead, our brains switch back and forth, albeit quickly, between the tasks in hand, leading to that mind-numbing feeling we know so well. They've also found that, far from being an efficient way to do things, we're more productive when we commit to doing just one thing at a time, one after the other – it takes *less* time to do that than it does to try to master all the things, all at once. When we attempt to multi-task, what we're really doing is battering our brain and draining it of its energy reserves. In overloading and overheating our cognitive abilities, we're putting ourselves under undue pressure and stress.

We also know, on some level, that multi-tasking doesn't work because we never feel as though our work is done; we never make it to the 'kick back and relax stage' of our day. Instead we end the day frazzled and frustrated because our to-do lists seem to mushroom throughout the day rather than shrink. Once we do make it to bed at night, it's not with a sense of accomplishment; it's with all the things we didn't get to do whizzing around our minds. We're wired and tired; that irritating state of unrest at the exact point we desperately need some shut-eye.

When our to-do lists are the length of our arms, and then some, it feels as though multi-tasking is the *only* way. It's certainly what we're used to and we know how our brains don't like change. But then, our brains don't like multi-tasking, either. We're darned if we do and darned if we don't.

Fret not: we have options. We always have options. Firstly, we can sack off the things we're doing out of a skewed sense of duty, the things that perhaps snuck in because our boundaries were wonky. We know the ones; the things looming in

'Multi-tasking doesn't work.'

our calendars that we're already trying to back out of. Just back out. We're allowed to change our minds, we're allowed to choose ourselves, we're allowed to make the right decisions for us and our families.

Hopefully, too, we'll have stretched the time available to us by clocking off work and by reducing the time we're on our smartphones.

And then we have the joy of batching! Batching is when we group tasks of a similar nature back to back. We do this without noticing already: we don't brush one tooth now and come back later to do another; we brush them all at the same time. We don't visit a supermarket umpteen times to fill our cupboards product by product; we tend to do a big shop all in one go.

Batching tasks can also help minimise decision fatigue. Rather than plan our meals each day, we can plan (and even prepare them) in one go, once a week. We can do the same thing with planning our outfits for the week ahead, with housework, with errands, when we're buying birthday cards, dealing with finances, responding to emails or social media notifications.

Time isn't the only valuable commodity that's stolen when we multi-task; we strain and drain our brains too.

Make Self-Care Non-Negotiable

There are things in life we just wouldn't do even if our lives depended on it. Those are our non-negotiables and they align with our core values. There's not a negotiator in the land who could sway us on those things. They're not even up for negotiation. The very thought of crossing those 'lines' sends us into a tailspin.

Yet we constantly compromise who we are. We cross the 'line' every day with our health when we don't allow time to recover from the stresses and strains of life. We demand so much of ourselves that we run the well dry. We sideline our needs until 'some' day, and 'some' day just never arrives. It's a mirage, an optical illusion, the lie we buy into. It's only when life has karate-chopped us to the floor that the penny drops. Then, and only then, does self-care become the tool we reach for.

We wouldn't treat anything else of value in such a shoddy way, which means we must be failing to see the value in who we are. Here's the thing: we matter because everybody matters. We're as worthy of life, laughter and love as the next person. We can't swap ourselves for someone else, so we might as well roll up our sleeves and vow to make the most of who we are and embrace the truth of who we are, no matter what our starting point may be.

It may be unchartered territory but self-care *is* non-negotiable and here's why: it deters ill health from our door, it's the simplifying of life, not the sacrificing of ourselves, the light to the dark, the pause in the go-go-go. It's our rehab from the demands of life, the self-permission to bloom, the regaining of control, the nemesis to burnout, the straightening of the skew-whiff, the blossoming friendship with ourselves, the release of tension, the nurturing of dreams, the redirection of energy, and an emphatic goodbye to the shoulds, coulds and buts.

We all deserve a big dollop of that.

Make Every Day a Self-Care Day

If our actions speak louder than our words, then our self-care actions might just quieten the thoughts we have about being unworthy and unimportant. The positive and intentional action will eventually negate the negative thoughts and feelings.

When we make every day a self-care day, we cultivate the new habit in a non-intrusive way. We're not asking ourselves to block out an hour a day (not yet, anyway . . . we can build up to that *wink wink*), we're looking for those micro pockets of time where we check in with ourselves, ponder how we're feeling, consider our energy levels, and act accordingly. Self-care is as much about the 'being' as it is the 'doing'. When we have the space to be, we can see more clearly what we might need to do to feel better.

That's why the #365daysofselfcare hashtag is so powerful. It's a nifty little hashtag, used predominantly on Twitter and Instagram, by people who have committed to an act of self-care every single day of the year. The hashtag brings up a plethora of self-care ideas as well as a community of people who are supportive of one another. It's a great way to chart progress and hold ourselves accountable, too. The hashtag also illustrates the kaleidoscope of ways our needs differ and can provide ideas for some self-care experimentation.

Planning space for self-care into our days gives us the benefit of foreseeing obstacles that might throw us off course. The slots we plan in aren't buffer times for chores and tasks to infringe upon; they're dedicated intervals to help us to feel better – whatever that may look like for each of us.

What 'self-care' acts are taking your fancy?
1
2
3
4
5

How will you make time for them?
1
2
3
4
5

Quick! Pop them into your calendar/schedule.

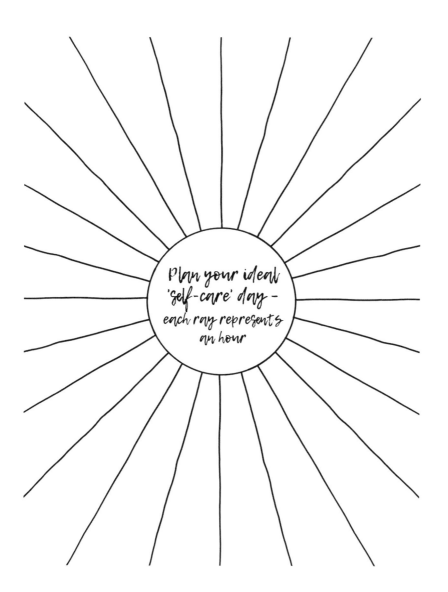

Plan your ideal 'self-care' day – each ray represents an hour

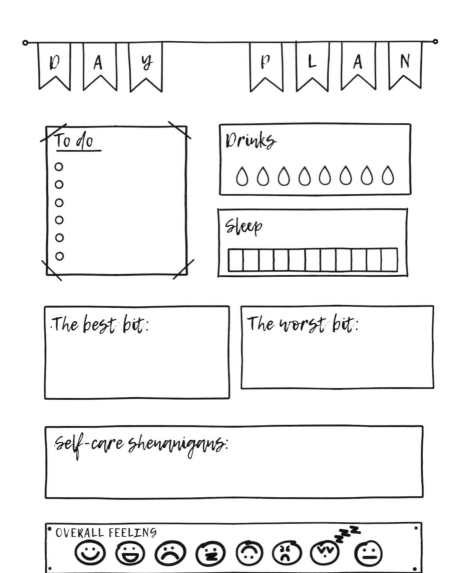

DAY PLAN

To do

- ○
- ○
- ○
- ○
- ○
- ○

Drinks

Sleep

The best bit:

The worst bit:

Self-care shenanigans:

OVERALL FEELING

8. A self-care squad: how it helps and what to do if we've not got one

'Who we surround ourselves with matters.'

An aspect of self-care that we don't always consider is the people we choose to spend our time with, the effect they can have on how our lives pan out, the effect we can have on how their lives pan out, and the effect that *not* having people to spend time with can have on our health and happiness.

Our opinions, thoughts, feelings, beliefs and behaviours are shaped, both directly and indirectly, by the people we spend time with. And the influence might not always be a favourable one. We're different people when left to our own devices than we are when we're surrounded by others – we tend to adopt the group mentality when we're with our friends.

Peer pressure and peer influence are associated with teenagers egging each other on to take part in something that might be frowned upon by their caregivers. What we don't realise is that the influence of our peers never goes away; we don't outgrow it, we don't become immune to it – it's part and parcel of our lives, whether that be a conscious influence we feel, or an unconscious one.

The structure of our schooling paves the way for quality time with our friends, every single term-time day (not to mention the hours we dedicate to speaking to our friends on the phone outside school hours). The sum of our responsibilities as young people is pretty much school work, friendships, and navigating the ever-changing physical and emotional landscape to adulthood. The paths we walk with those school friends are often parallel in their nature and their experiences: lessons, homework, bands we listen to, magazines and books we read, exams, puberty, and the self-discovery process. We put a lot of time, energy and commitment into maintaining, fostering and prioritising those friendships.

Fast-forward five, ten, fifteen years into full-blown adulthood and many of those friendships will have petered out, our paths having meandered in different directions. Our friendships become vulnerable due to circumstance and don't always stand the test of time. Our adult selves have additional responsibilities to consider and juggle, and more demands on our time for those friendships to compete with: romantic relationships, work, bills, children, pets, living in different geographical areas, breakdown of family units, illness. The time we have available for our friendships is reduced considerably and unless we make time for those friendships, they sadly fall by the wayside.

Who we surround ourselves with matters. It matters because friendships form the basis of our support squad; the complex network of people with whom we have a relationship, through choice. Those we give and receive support from.

It matters because of the peer influence aspect; people can elevate us, inspire us, encourage us, root for us and help us realise our goals. People can also drain us, undermine us, be the source of conflict and rivalry, hold us back, affect our self-confidence and bring untoward drama to our lives.

It matters because those people influence our decisions, our actions, our thoughts and our feelings. We're more influenced by others than we think we are.

Success, in our self-care plans, and anything else, can be helped greatly by the people we have around us.

Some key squad positions might be:

The Encourager

We all need an encourager in life; a person with a big heart who shakes their pom-poms, cheers us on, roots for us, who has an unwavering belief in us. They understand what's important to us, buy into our dreams, and make us feel capable of anything.

When we're racked with self-doubt and have listed all the reasons why we can't do something, they'll kindly walk us through all the reasons we can, and will.

Their energy and outlook is infectious; we leave their company feeling buoyed up, lit up, more confident and as though anything is possible.

The Encourager will be the first to celebrate the good times

'Success, in our self-care plans, and anything else, can be helped greatly by the people we have around us.'

with us, but will equally be there at the drop of a hat to help us through the dark by magnifying hope and courage.

The Inspiring One

When we're inspired, we feel called to act, to stand tall and to stand up for what we believe in. It's the fire we feel in the pit of our stomachs that compels us to do something.

That 'something' can be anything: to follow our dreams, to keep going through the tough times, to campaign, to vote, to petition, to write, to be whatever we want to be and do whatever we want to do.

When we're surrounded by inspiring people, we can't help but get swept along by their energy. They don't just break through glass ceilings, they smash through them – obstacles, shobstacles. Blueprint, what blueprint? They carve their own way, refusing to be labelled or pigeon-holed. As our friends, they're generous in the sharing of their experiences too; they share the nitty-gritty of their hardships and they're happy to answer questions about how they overcome them.

They seem to be at ease with who they are because they 'own' their vulnerabilities, in that they're very aware of them and happy to talk about them, but they won't let those vulnerabilities hold them back.

The Clown

The morale-boosting, quirky, good-natured, funny friend who has us giggling like a snorting hyena.

Time flies when we're with this one and we always leave feeling lighter and with a stitch in our side from all the laughter. They bring out our funny side, keep us grounded, and we look forward to the banter, in jokes and rapport.

Far from being superficial, these friends simply magnify the lighter side of life. We feel safe in their company because we know they'll never overstep the mark with their humour; we're not the butt of their jokes, we're just 'in' on the joke.

Laughter is a tonic and it flows freely when we're with this friend. It's never forced – they don't even need to try to be funny; they just are, and we feel as though we're funnier when we're with them.

The Empathiser

They just get 'it', whatever 'it' is. We feel understood, cared for and heard when we're with these friends. They laugh with us and they cry with us, having the innate knack of relating to our pain.

We know we've spent time with an empathetic ear because we've opened up with ease, spoken of our vulnerabilities and pain, and felt a deep connection, with zero judgement and criticism. Being with them is like being wrapped in a gigantic duvet; we feel safe, validated and held.

Wonderfully perceptive, too, at times the Empathiser will play devil's advocate, allowing us a window into a different perspective.

The Challenger

We're wholly responsible for our actions but when we share our goals with our friends, they can help us to remain on the path towards those goals.

The Challenger will do their best to keep us committed; they'll question our actions and decisions if it seems we're digressing, and ask any other questions that need asking. They help us to get out of our own way.

There's a level of trust and confidentiality that we hold dear with these friends.

Erm ...
  Hold up a minute ...
  What about those of us who find ourselves alone, isolated and squad-less?

Friendships don't always come easily; they can be tricky beasts. Perhaps we've always found it difficult to gel with others, perhaps our friendships didn't stand the test of time, perhaps our friendships have been damaged beyond repair, perhaps they've cracked and need mending but nobody is making the first move, maybe mental ill health saw us emotionally withdrawing from friendships or highlighted the cracks that were already there. It could be that our friendships just gradually faded into those of acquaintances.

Sometimes we find ourselves adrift, alone and isolated. This might be because we're away from home, a relationship has broken down, we're in the middle of a storm of conflict, unemployed, working from home, because we have mobility issues, or we might be emotionally isolated due to illness.

We can feel isolated and alone when we haven't seen or spoken with anyone for periods of time but we can feel alone when we're surrounded by other people too, especially when we feel misunderstood or uncared for. *Being* alone isn't the same as *feeling* alone. Sometimes we genuinely do enjoy, and need, our own space.

When we feel alone – whether that's a fleeting feeling, a prolonged feeling, or due to the situation we're in – it hurts. It hurts a lot. It's distressing and painful because it makes space for those negative thoughts to breed like wild rabbits; those nasty thoughts that tell us that we're hopeless, helpless, unlikeable, that something must be inherently wrong with us to end up so alone and that nobody would miss us if we were to disappear.

With nobody to fight our corner or to challenge our negative perspective on ourselves, we become locked in a vicious circle – one that damages our mental and physical health. We end up feeling nervous about social interactions; we think twice about them, avoid them, convinced that we have nothing to offer but at the same time feeling increasingly awkward, scared of rejection and calling our social skills into question. This vicious circle dents our already knocked confidence further, which in turn keeps us lonely.

We don't always link the two but chronic loneliness is a health-related matter; we're wired to thrive when we feel supported, connected and on the receiving end of empathy. When we lack the social connection we need, our health is affected. Loneliness contributes to cognitive decline, affects our longevity, puts our immune system under strain, disturbs our sleep and increases the risk of stress-related illnesses.

It's frightening.

It takes buckets of courage, self-kindness and discipline to break this cycle but there are things we can do to break free from it. Nobody deserves to be alone, despite what the negative thoughts are telling us. Bearing the brunt of self-blame and beating ourselves up are sure-fire ways of keeping us in the cycle that we so desperately would like to escape from. Here are some ways to help us do just that:

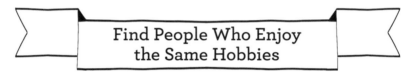

Find People Who Enjoy the Same Hobbies

It's easier to foster a connection with someone when there's an established common interest; it takes the focus away from the small talk and foregoes the need to be a great conversation-starter. There are organised groups for all sorts of hobbies – common and niche, both online and offline. Whether you fancy revisiting an old hobby that you once enjoyed, giving a new one a go or learning a new skill, classes, clubs and groups can be a fantastic shortcut to making new friends and building on the natural shared-interest foundation of friendship.

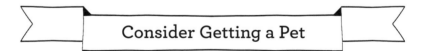

Consider Getting a Pet

If it's feasible to do so and you don't mind the responsibility that comes with it, getting a pet such as a cat or dog is a two-pronged approach to reducing isolation and loneliness. In addition to the unconditional love and companionship our pets provide, they kick-start conversations with other pet owners. If getting a pet isn't an option, then we can offer to walk our neighbour's dog or even sign up to borrowmydoggy.com and look after someone else's.

Embrace the Community Aspect of Social Media

Social media provides us with a window onto the outside world but it can also contribute to our sense of detachment and make us feel worse about our current circumstances. It's how it makes us feel that determines whether it's an act of self-care for us to dive in, or not.

And that's the best bit about social media platforms – we can dip in and out when it suits us. We can also follow people with common interests and interact with them – it sometimes feels more comfortable reaching out to start a conversation with a stranger online than it does face-to-face. Facebook has groups that were started to help bring together people who are facing a similar problem and harness support from our peers; there are groups for those who are lonely, groups for those who have a mental illness, groups for those who are grieving, and so many more.

Join, or Start, a Meetup

Meetup.com is an amazing network of thousands of local events/ groups. If you have a hobby, or are facing a problem, then Meetup will almost certainly have an event/group for you. There are groups for runners, crafters, writers, board game players, film nights, surfing, book clubs, people who are working together on social and political campaigns, people who are lonely, people who are shy, anxiety support, depression support, cancer support . . . and if the group we are looking for isn't there, we can start our own.

Volunteer

There are organisations across the world who are crying out for help, and volunteering our time to those organisations is how they're able to help more people. Volunteering is as beneficial to the volunteer as it is to the organisation. In facilitating and furthering the work of some amazing social causes, we can welcome personal benefits such as being introduced to new experiences, gaining new skills and qualifications, developing a sense of purpose, cultivating friendships, opening the door for a new career, and boosting our confidence.

Start a Blog

A blog is a corner of the internet which is all ours; we get to decide what we write, when we write it and how much creativity we want to pour into it. They're free and relatively simple to set up, too. There are blogs on all manner of topics – all we have to do is decide what we'd like to write about and get writing. A blog can work as an outlet for our thoughts, act as a diary charting our progress in a personal goal or hobby, or it can simply be a collection of our favourite things. There's a sense of pride we feel when we build something that matters to us. 'Build it and they will come' has never been truer of the blogging community; there will be people who are really interested in what we have to say and it's a great way to find our tribe, build a community of our own, and connect with people from all over the world.

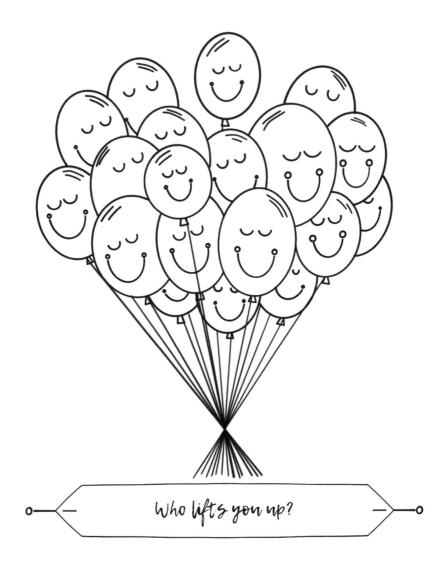

Who lifts you up?

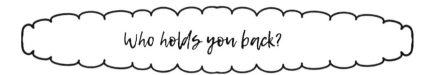

Who holds you back?

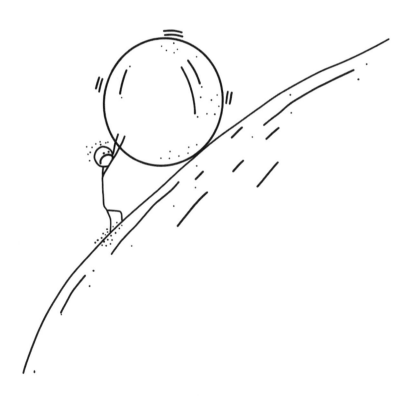

What's missing? What support do you need?

_____
_____
_____

_____
_____
_____

_____
_____
_____

_____
_____
_____

9. What to do when our self-care mojo disappears (because it will)

'Maintaining motivation is a continual work in progress.'

Wahoo! We've got this self-care malarkey nailed; we've been doing it for weeks and we're shimmying through life with an almighty spring in our step. We can't believe it took us so long to get started! We're triumphant and proud.

Then one day we wake up and for no apparent reason, we've hit a brick wall. The honeymoon period is well and truly over. We're discouraged. The sinking feeling in our stomach has returned and is playing havoc with our carefully laid plans.

Self-care is a challenge again.

Oh.

We didn't see this coming . . .

Mojo, or motivation, is a b-e-a-utiful thing. When we're motivated, we feel energised, full of get-up-and-go, driven, inspired, enthused and fulfilled. When we start something that we're highly motivated to start, it's a doddle.

But when the initial euphoric wave of motivation wanes, it's quite another story.

Motivation can be a slippery eel; in our grasp one moment, only to have disappeared out of sight the next. It's a given that our motivation will go AWOL from time to time; motivation ebbs and flows and life's disruptive nature means that we need to consciously recharge our motivation. When our get-up-and-go has got up and gone, there's a sense of detachment, frustration and despondency; we feel stuck in a rut. Everything feels harder than it used to. We've run out of steam.

Losing our motivation isn't as simple as 'it's lost and we need to find it'. Our motivation can falter for any number of reasons. Expecting that it will falter is one half of the battle. The other half is allowing space for mindfulness to help us isolate the source of the current bout of funk so we can nurture motivation's comeback.

Maintaining motivation is a continual work in progress. If we can identify why (doesn't it always come back to our 'why'?!) it went away, then we can understand where to find it so we can make strides to bolster it again.

We're Overloaded

If we've simply added self-care on top of all the other things we've got going on for us, rather than making time for it as an 'instead of', then we can topple from the sheer weight of it all.

Motivation can be the rocket fuel that leads us to achieve remarkable things; it's what helps us to feel super-human, as though we can take on the world. And we can, one step at a time. Motivation propels us, it gives us that extra oomph; it can also add a sense of urgency that leads us to take on too much, too soon. In our keenness we find we've gone all 'hell, yeah!' to too many things at once, perhaps bitten off more than we can chew.

It's a quick-fire way of draining our motivation battery.

When we're overwhelmed, stressed, tired and depleted, our motivation has already left the building. It's tempting to keep going, to push harder in the hope that motivation will return, but it rarely does and is more likely to lead to burnout.

The good news? The seed for motivation is still there, our interest is still piqued, but we've simply set off out of the starting blocks a little rambunctiously, and it's quite likely that our self-confidence has taken a knock in the process.

It's important to stop, just for a spell. To take time to strip back, to simplify where we can, to slow down the tempo and give ourselves the chance to recalibrate. It's also time to reflect on how far we've come. When we constantly look ahead at where we want to be, we rarely allow ourselves to bathe in the glory of our progress. Once we get to where we want to be, we're inclined to move the goalposts, to strive for

'It's important to stop, just for a spell.'

more, to challenge ourselves further – but it's equally important to celebrate our growth and pat ourselves on the back. Our past experiences can also teach us some valuable lessons, which only become clear with hindsight, which, in turn, is only achieved through contemplation

We're Scared

Our old friend (or foe?) fear is doing a number on us. Just when we thought we had this stuff sussed, fear taps us on the shoulder and asks, 'Are you *sure* this is what you want?' It's a trick question, loaded with self-doubt, insecurity and a lack of self-confidence.

Fear can be a tremendous motivator but it can also stop motivation in its tracks quick-smart.

There will, of course, be times when fear is our greatest ally, but those times are few and far between because it's not often (well, we certainly hope not) that we're in great danger and the fight-or-flight instinct is relevant. When we're motivated by fear, we are powered by adrenaline, by our inbuilt capacity to survive. We're motivated by what we don't want to happen and it spurs us on. It can be a fraught sort of motivation, one that isn't always considered or planned. It's instinctive; it's primal.

Fear can, of course, keep us safe, but it doesn't half hold us back too, initiating the fight-or-flight instinct when it's just so unnecessary. Fear can stun us and keep us where we are. It's the inbuilt tool we have for weighing up perceived risks. When the fear siren kicks in, we start to doubt the way forward and start to doubt ourselves.

Fear can become a gigantic roadblock, blocking us from the extraordinary. This is when it weakens us, momentarily.

But when we're venturing into unknown territory, fear is a constant companion, the thorn in our side. It never goes away, we just learn to size it up and to carry on regardless. Each small step (with 'small' being the operative word here) we take alongside fear, the stronger we eventually grow.

We're at a Fork in The Road

We've been pootling along and suddenly we're faced with a decision – not a little decision, but a mighty one that could change the course of our lives.

Not knowing which way to turn, we've spent a considerable amount of time listing the reasons for and against each option, we've played devil's advocate until we're blue in the face, we've called in the opinions of everyone and their dog, and we've covered all angles in infinitesimal detail. We're still stumped.

The collection of data we've accumulated hasn't helped. Not in the least. If anything, it's heightened the indecision and confusion. We're well and truly stuck. Motivation is sitting in the wings until a decision has been made.

Groundhog Day.

Delegating the decision is a rubbish back-up plan, too; it just gives us someone to blame should it all go wrong. It disempowers us. We can draw on the experiences and insights of others but ultimately the decision, and responsibility, is ours.

When we find ourselves dithering in this way, it's often because we lack clarity about what we want the result to be. Caught in the moment, in feeling lost, we forget the big picture: Does either of these options lead us towards, or away from our dreams? What is the outcome we're aiming for? Does either of these choices lead us there?

If we can buy ourselves some time to get clear on that, then the path will usually present itself. It might be that neither option supports the outcome we're after and that's okay too. Making *no* decision can be a decision in itself if it's intentional and not a form of procrastination.

If nothing feels right, then maybe, just maybe, there's another option waiting to be discovered.

We've Changed

When we tune into how we feel (the basis of self-care), we become more and more aware of how interchangeable those feelings can be. The ever-changing landscape calls for flexibility and tweaks.

What was right for us once won't always be right for us. We change, we evolve and we grow. What once motivated us might not serve as a motivator any longer. Those motivators might now be defunct.

There are two things we can be sure of: life is fleeting and change is inevitable. Each day that we're held ransom by others (and sometimes ourselves) to remain the same is a day less that we have left to live life the way we would choose to. Changing our minds does not mean that we're flaky or unreliable. We do not need to apologise for who we are.

Life is a transformative process; it's intended to be that way. From the day we are born, until the day we die, we have access to new experiences, new perspectives, new cultures, new people and new lessons.

'We're allowed to change our minds, to change direction.'

We're allowed to change our minds, to change direction, to outgrow relationships, to do a U-turn on thoughts and beliefs, to tear up someone else's rulebook, to forge our own paths, to shake off the expectations and limitations of others, to amend the terms, to experiment, to step into our power. We're allowed to be different; not just in how we're different from others but also in how we may have been before. Much as we're allowed to remain the same, if that's what we choose to do.

If our motivators no longer serve us, some motivator maintenance is called for; space to reflect on what's changed and what needs to change, to re-evaluate our commitment to rooted habits and to find a new equilibrium, *should* do the trick.

We're Doing It For The Wrong Reasons

There may be times we find ourselves in a lousy predicament: motivated for all the wrong reasons. This is the hardest motivation to foster because it most likely didn't come from within in the first place. It's akin to trying to jumpstart a car that has the wrong battery; we're not going to get very far.

That motivation can come from a sense of obligation; we're doing things because we feel we ought to (that blasted Law of Should, again) and not because we necessarily want to.

With self-care, this is typically when we haven't spent the time getting to grips with our needs and have adopted the self-care practices of other people. We've just followed suit. It feels icky from the get-go.

In trying to keep up with the Joneses, we're motivated by tenuous yardsticks based on other people's measures of success and not based on what's important to us at our core. Motivation is as fleeting as the material goods by which we're defining power, success and values.

When motivation is bred from manipulation or pressure from others, we feel as though our hands have been forced and as though we're living a lie. We're uncomfortable, we're full of resentment and we're reluctant to continue.

Shamed-based motivation comes from a nasty place; it plays into our fear, our perceived flaws and our anxiety. We may be motivated by shame when we've been humiliated and feel as though we're defective in some way. It isn't sustainable without further damage to our self-esteem, our confidence and our sense of identity.

There are times, too, when motivation can be infectious – it sweeps us along on its wave. When the initial enthusiasm fades, we sometimes find ourselves unwittingly in tricky situations that we want to back out of because the motivation wasn't ours to begin with.

When motivation has done a runner in these circumstances, it's a red flag that tells us that our heart's not in it, that our actions are out of whack with our values – we might as well follow suit and do a runner from those situations too.

We Might Be Depressed

What if we don't remember the last time we felt motivated to do anything? What if, however much we try to force it, with all the tricks of the trade, motivation remains elusive? What if it feels as though we're walking through treacle? What if our brain just won't play ball?

Depression is a debilitating mental illness which affects every aspect of our lives. The symptoms vary in their severity and are not limited to feeling hopeless, helpless and unworthy. Exhaustion, irritability, a foggy head, numbness, no interest in the things that once brought us pleasure, emotional withdrawal from loved ones, sleeping difficulties, limited energy, increased anxiety over answering the phone, making decisions and opening the post, altered sex drive, change in appetite and inescapable thoughts which can sometimes lead to self-harm and suicide.

It's an insidious illness, creeping into our every thought, every action, every movement. It's much more than sadness or a bad spell. It is a conveyor belt of shifting emotions and feelings; of being super-aware of our surroundings yet numb to them; of craving love and acceptance but rejecting them; of having a brain that doesn't stop but which also doesn't quite seem to work; it's caring too much and caring not at all. It's the Herculean effort to get out of bed. The enormity of tasks we once undertook on autopilot. It's the loudness of the world mixed with the loudness of the thoughts that make us wish for a mute button. It's not an illness we can just snap out of, however hard we try. We also can't be shamed out of it, forced out of it or bullied out

'Self-care is depression's nemesis.'

'Every micro action of self-care is a way to stick two fingers up to depression.'

of it. It just doesn't work in that way.

The gap between where we are and where other people appear to be is a precipitous chasm. It feels unnavigable too.

It's difficult to care for someone, to nurture them, when we don't like them. That's what depression does to us – it robs us of our identity and plays us off against ourselves. There's a sense of futility to self-care, as though we're fighting a losing battle and biding our time until it ends.

But self-care is depression's nemesis. There's no doubt about that.

It's not in depression's interest that we take care of ourselves because it diminishes depression's power and control. When we feel so out of control, it's the tiny actions of self-care that give us control, however briefly. They show depression that, no matter how tentative our grasp, we still have hold of the reins; that we're in charge. Self-care shows depression that who we are still exists despite depression's overwhelming presence. When actions of self-care compound, they become the basis from which our strength grows, our hope grows and our sense of identity rebuilds. Every micro action of self-care is a way to stick two fingers up to depression; it's a micro battle won even when the odds feel stacked against us. We must never forget: we're enough, as we are, even when unwell. We've absolutely got what it takes to be victorious over depression. We can do this and we *will* do this. At a snail's pace, yes, but undoubtedly, surely.

Consider this: what advice would your elder-self
give you right now? Pop it in the box below.

That older self of yours is a wise 'ol owl

Make a list of the things that comfort
you on lemon-pelting days

○

○

○

○

○

○

○

○

○

○

My self-care declaration

I promise to:

_____

I will remember to:

_____

At all times, particularly in times of
stress or uncertainty, I will:

_____

_____

I will try my absolute hardest to:

_____

I will choose kindness. Always.

Signed: _____ .

10. Emergency self-care

There will be times when life knocks us to our knees and we don't have headspace to consider what might help. Here are some suggestions of self-care activites which may help in these 'emergency' self-care situations.

Self-Care When We Crave Comfort

We're told that the magic happens outside our comfort zone, but what about the magic that occurs inside our comfort zone?

There are times when we're grieving, have lost a loved one or are experiencing pain, and have been making so many changes outside our comfort zone, when being inside our comfort zone is exactly the place we need to be for a bit.

There's something to be said for the nurturing, reassuring safety of comfort, for stepping off the treadmill of life. It soothes us back to strength, gives us space to take stock and allows tension to dissipate. We're going to batten down the hatches, place a 'do not disturb' sign on the door, switch our phones to airplane mode, and make a comfort retreat.

How to create the ultimate comfort retreat

1 WARMTH
A retreat isn't a retreat without some warmth to calm and nourish us. There's something satisfying about hunkering down into warmth. Hot-water bottles, a warm bubble bath, blankets, duvets, furry friends, clean bedding, a hot drink, some warm woolly socks and an oversized sweater all bring that warm, fuzzy feeling.

2 ESCAPISM
The realities of life aren't always pleasant. The boredom, the fear, the pain can all get a bit much. Wanting to escape from it, understanding full well that we'll have to return to it at some point, is normal. We all feel this way at times; we want to step away from reality and be distracted. Forget about your problem, just for a while, by losing yourself in a book, a movie, some comedy or a video game.

3 BRAIN-DUMP
Having a notebook and pen nearby gives us an outlet to brain-dump our worries but also to capture any ideas or solutions that pop up.

4 BAKE
The smell of home-baked goodness, the process, the nostalgia, the tasting . . .

5 CREATE AMBIENCE
Whatever surrounds us and taps into our senses can alter the way we feel. A comforting atmosphere can be made quite quickly using scented candles, fairy lights, pillow and room spray, diffusers and flowers.

6 SEEK COMFORT
Sometimes the comfort we seek is the comfort of others. It can help to share worries with someone we trust, whether the aim of that is to seek advice, to offload or to brain-dump. The people we seek comfort from might not always be friends, either; they might come in the form of professionals, such as the Samaritans.

Self-care for when life pelts lemons at us

We've all had 'those' days which have rolled into two, maybe three, possibly a week, a month, a year – a stretch of time when it feels as though life is just pelting lemons at us, repeatedly. A chaotic patch of life which tests our resolve to the limit. Everything that could go wrong does go wrong. We're beyond stressed. We're at our wits' end. Kerplunked.

Problem solving takes brainpower, courage and resilience. It's hard to pick ourselves up again, and again, and again.

The knee-jerk reaction is to keep ploughing on but it rarely all goes away without a re-steering of the ship:

1 FOSTER SELF-BELIEF
Dealing with problem after problem is wearing; it grinds us down and, depending on our life experiences, we might not feel equipped to deal with them.

We've got this – we *so* have. It doesn't feel like it, as all the plates are spinning out of control, or crashing, but we have what it takes to get through this.

We've been through rough patches before and got through them, even when we didn't believe we would.

The odd thing about problems is that the more of them we deal with, the more equipped our future selves will feel to deal with the obstacles that come our way. It's one of the cruel jokes of life; overcoming problems increases our self-confidence and our resilience.

2 PLAY TO THE SENSES

Whilst we're being ninja problem-sorter-outers, we're putting our energy and brainpower to the test. It's important that we take time out from our ninja-ing to refill those tanks, to catch a breath and to rest up.

Problems always feel bigger than they are when we're smack-bang in the middle of them. We desperately search for the solution only for it to present itself when we're doing something completely unrelated; cooking our dinner, reading a book or taking a shower. When we give ourselves space from the problem, we give our brains a chance to digest it, to join the dots and come up with a solution. Our brains will work for us, if only we give them a chance.

We can give our frazzled brains a well-earned break if we employ the help of our senses, too; light a scented candle, go outside and smell some flowers, run a bath, snuggle up in blankets, have a delicious snack, listen to some music, watch a film, breathe in some fresh air.

3 SEARCH FOR THE OPPORTUNITY

Problems can loom larger than life and they can be a downright nuisance. Our brains prefer the known to the unknown. When the unknown is thrust into our face, we freeze and self-doubt floods in.

A P45 signals the end of employment and probably the end of our bill-paying income. It could also end the spell of working a job we hate, of having to jump through hoops to keep a grouchy boss happy, or a long commute. What's it the beginning of? Every beginning is preceded by the ending of something else.

Sometimes breakdown precedes breakthrough. Sometimes all these lemons are highlighting the ducks that are out of their row. Sometimes the problems are teaching us something important. Sometimes we just need to ride the storm and wait for the epic karma party that's on its way.

4 ONE THING AT A TIME

When everything is going wrong at the same time, we naturally want to fix it all at the same time. When everything is screaming for our attention, we're not sure which way to turn first; we're in a tailspin.

We can start by getting some sort of order to our thoughts, problems and tasks. Brain-dump everything that's taking up valuable headspace – everything. The things that are urgent, the things that are important, the problems, the tasks, the chores, the obligations and the wants. On a blank page, we can then start prioritising these things, with self-care at the very top. Taking time for self-care will rejuvenate us to keep going. By slicing and dicing this very long list, we can group together the things that are urgent, the things that are important, the things we can delegate, the things we can forget about, the things we need to back out of and the things we need help with, and then act accordingly.

5 STOP

It always feels wrong to stop when life is forcing you to live in the fast lane. It goes against all the instincts and pressure we feel. Pressing pause is an action, in and of itself. Turbulence doesn't bring clarity; it's by having the courage to stop, when the world is at its most demanding, that clarity, peace and revelation are found.

Self-Care for Exhausted New Parents

We wrestle with time for self-care pre-parenthood but there's no time-shrinker quite like having a baby.

There's no denying it, being a new parent is a jungle of emotions, experiences and lessons.

Well-meaning advice pings at us from many angles and it can be so contradictory. Added to that is a teeny weeny little 'un who is depending on us for all their needs to be met – 24/7. We're novices and don't we know it. The uncertainty, the weight of responsibility, sleepless nights and the winging-it factor make for an exhausting combination. There's so much to get our heads around.

It feels harder than ever, but it's now more important than ever to make sure our needs are met so that we're strong enough to bear the weight of this new miraculous-but-still-intimidating responsibility.

1 SELF-FORGIVENESS

We set our expectations of what our parenting style will be like long before baby arrives and we tend to set it wayyyyy high. We don't account for the internal tug-of-war, the quadrupled chores, the vomit, the sheer quantity of nappies, the goodness knows what that's dried into our top, the one-armed shuffle as we try to do anything with baby asleep in our arms, the curveballs.

There isn't a parent in the land who hasn't at times felt inadequate, out of their depth, tired to the core, tested and exasperated. Just as we won't shout at our children when they're learning to walk and stumble, we mustn't beat ourselves up as we're learning to parent and stumble. We're on a grizzly learning curve which is physically and emotionally draining. When we pick fault with ourselves, we're not allowing room for growth or learning; we're instead wasting the very little energy we have on things we probably won't remember even happened when we're further down the line. We do our best and that's all anyone, including ourselves, can ask of us.

2 ASK FOR SPACE IF YOU NEED IT

There's nothing like the promise of a cuddle with a newborn to have all and sundry flocking to our homes. The last thing we feel like doing as new parents is sprucing ourselves up for visitors and making our homes presentable. We're knackered. We need sleep. But our politeness often prevents us from saying 'no' to home visits and we can easily find ourselves a little overwhelmed and intruded upon.

The tidal wave of messages and visit requests come from a good place; these people are excited and delighted that parents and baby are doing well – that still doesn't make it any easier to deal with. Especially if family politics are involved.

If it all feels a little much, then we need to lay down some boundaries and have a strategy in place. Give priority to those you don't mind wearing pyjamas in front of (they're usually the people we can be ourselves around) and postpone the rest. Their time will come.

3 ASK FOR HELP

They say it takes a village to raise a child but what if we don't have a village? What if we've found ourselves navigating this landscape alone or as a tiny team? What if the support we expected to have just isn't there? What if we're not coping at all?

As with everything in life, knowing someone has our back boosts our emotional and physical wellbeing.

The support we receive as new parents typically comes from our partner, our friends and our family (if we're lucky enough to have those). Health visitors are also on hand to support parents and baby. If either parent feels as though they aren't receiving enough support, are experiencing symptoms of depression or have questions, then the health visitor would be the first port of call. They're the gateway to lots of other sources of assistance, too: doctors, support groups (both online and offline), community groups, helplines, counsellors and other resources.

It's never easy to ask for help but the sooner we do, the quicker it comes. And we deserve it, we really do.

4 ACCEPT HELP

We don't like accepting help at the best of times; we don't want to put other people out, we don't like feeling vulnerable, as though we're not coping, and we're never quite sure if the 'let me know if I can do anything to help' comments are sincere.

It takes time to adjust to being a parent, to flex to the changing needs of your baby and for a routine, of sorts, to be established.

Offers of assistance do tend to come from a place of empathy, an understanding that our lives have been turned upside down and that we might need some assistance. Or, at the very least, a breather – a shower, a hot drink and a tasty meal – we'll have plenty of chances to acclimatise to lukewarm tea later (it's an acquired taste)!

People genuinely like to help and we're not asking for the earth. If the roles were reversed, we totally wouldn't mind cuddling a newborn whilst the parents had a shower, we wouldn't mind bringing a dish of casserole so that the parents just need to reheat it to eat, and we absolutely wouldn't mind picking up some groceries on our way over.

Accepting help really does make a difference; it eases the pressure we feel and gives us some much-needed breathing room.

5 LEAVE COMPARISON WELL ALONE

When we embark down the road of comparing ourselves to others, we'd better be prepared for war – the war we're waging with ourselves. We've all been there and it never ever ends well.

We live in a world where we've ample opportunity to take a glimpse into the lives of others. Pretty much on demand.
The scenes we see aren't always as real as they seem; they might be filtered, cropped, staged. We just don't know. Yet, we take them at face value. We size ourselves up against those images and are left feeling pretty rotten about ourselves as a result. We question their choices, question our choices, compare their choices with our choices. Every child is different, every mother is different, every father is different; every situation is different. Nothing is as easy as it looks. Nobody has all the answers. We never fully know what's going on behind the scenes. When we compare another person's shining moments with our very worst bits, we're always going to fall short.

6 ALWAYS CHOOSE SLEEP

The sleep deprivation is relentless; there's no let-up. We go to put the milk in the bin and the tea towels in the fridge, and it's anyone's guess what our names are – we'll answer to anything at this point. We could sleep for days but, y'know, bubs needs feeding, soothing and nappy changing.

The fight for sleep is real and the impact that lack of sleep has on us is real too. It's a given that we probably won't manage our usual seven to nine hours, but we can make the most of the time we do have available to power nap.

Whenever possible, choose sleep. Choose sleep when baby sleeps, choose sleep over household chores, choose sleep over Facebook, choose sleep over Netflix, choose sleep over anything you can get away with because sleep is your friend. Ask friends to come over so you can sleep, tag team with your partner so you can sleep. Employ any means available to you to help you sleep: pillow spray, relaxation apps, soothing music, warm milk, black-out blinds, a sleep mask, chamomile tea . . .

And when we're overtired and sleep doesn't come easily, taking some quiet time out for a bath, to read a book and or to grab some fresh air can be restorative too.

Self-Care for When We're Empty and Have Nothing Left to Give

Sometimes we find ourselves on our knees; our motivation has deserted us, our energy tanks are depleted, we feel everything and nothing, all at once. We're empty. Bone dry.

This often brings with it a sense of frustration – 'Why can't I be more like [insert name of friend who is posting their achievements all over social media]?'

Guilt – 'I was supposed to be helping so-and-so with all the things.'

And shame – 'I could do XYZ with my eyes closed a year ago; now I can barely leave my bed.'

When we feel empty and as though we have nothing left to give, self-care is critical. It's also when it feels most impossible – the very time we have no headspace even to consider what might help us to feel better. We've been left with a foggy head, heavy heart and weary limbs and, to make matters worse, it feels as though the world is ganging up on us, wanting more, and more, and more.

The slant on self-care becomes more about survival, as rest-and-recovery mode is initiated. Everything else can, and must, wait.

Survival self-care is doing the bare minimum to get back on our feet. As well as making sure we are eating regularly and drinking enough fluid, here are some things that may help:

1 TAKE A NAP

It's not lazy to start paying back the sleep deficit we've no doubt built up juggling all those balls, it's really not. Sleep is an imperative part of our wellbeing. When we're asleep, our bodies can begin to heal. When we're struggling to sleep, try listening to soothing music or use a white noise app.

2 BE MINDFUL OF NEGATIVE SELF-TALK

When we're empty, we sometimes have a skewed perspective on ourselves yet see others with rose-tinted spectacles. It's divisive; it becomes about 'us and them'. We need to try to be our own best friend – to treat ourselves with the patience and kindness we would show to others. Our words can harm or heal.

3 CALL IN THE CAVALRY

Don't be afraid to ask for guidance. If a friend were in a similar situation, we'd jump to their aid. It's now our turn to do just that. Friends can assist with childcare, by preparing meals that we can chuck into the oven, by sitting with us when needed, by helping us to take care of bills, and by supporting us in whatever way we need them.

This also applies to other people who may be able to support us – support groups, helplines, doctors, self-help books – anyone who can help make life just that little bit easier. The more supported we are, the better.

4 RETREAT

Consider some time out from work, school, life. Channel our inner tortoise and take it slow, hibernate for a while, take comfort in our duvet and Netflix. Allow ourselves room to breathe and recover. It's important. Whilst we're at it, limiting social media is a good shout, too – we don't need to see the highlights and hustle when we're feeling so low. It's not a level playing field.

5 QUIETEN YOUR PHONE

Smartphones can be noisy and intrusive. Consider switching off all alerts – emails, social media, texts, voicemail, WhatsApp, etc. Rather than being demanded to check in because a flashing light/vibration tells us to, we can then mindfully check in when we choose to do so. It helps us to take back some control in a world where it's easy to feel as though we don't have any.

6 KEEP/MAKE THOSE DOCTOR'S APPOINTMENTS

Self-care is sometimes about doing the very things we have been procrastinating over. If there's something that's been bothering us health-wise, let's make that appointment. Take a friend for support. But go. Go now. The sooner we get checked out, the sooner our mind can be put to rest, or we can access professional help. It's a win-win.

7 SAY 'NO' MORE

Now is the time to say 'yes' to us. It's not easy to say 'no' to others when they're so used to hearing 'yes', but our wellbeing is our ultimate responsibility and can't be shelved any longer. Anything that makes us feel weighed down by others' expectations, resentful, frustrated and angry, is a down-and-out 'no'. An 'always no', too, not a 'not now' no.

8 CONSIDER WHAT WE ENJOYED AS A CHILD

As we get sucked into the 'being an adult' vortex, we forget to play – to do things simply because we enjoy them, for enjoyment's sake. Play dominates our time as children but is often non-existent as we grow older. Take inspiration from the things we enjoyed when we were children and see how we enjoy them now. We might rediscover some ways to unwind and distract.

9 START A JOURNAL

Our thoughts don't always make sense; they can be cruel, loud and ferocious. When we journal, we give those thoughts an outlet, somewhere else to be. In black and white, their power sometimes lessens. A journal can also help us to identify patterns in the way we are feeling – what might have caused those feelings when we feel our best and when we feel our worst. A journal can also serve as a real-time reminder of the progress we're making.

10 START A POSITIVITY JAR

Positivity may well grate on us right now, as it's so far from where we are – the negative thoughts might be in abundance with plenty of anecdotal evidence as to why we're helpless, hopeless and worthless. Those thoughts are lying, and so it's important to start collecting evidence against them – the nice things that people have said (whether we agree or not), the kind things people have done, the kind things we have done, the glimmers of hope in an otherwise dark time, our wins. Jot them down, keep them. Read back over them when a dose of sunshine is needed.

11 DECLUTTER

Our surroundings can affect the way we feel, and there's nothing quite as stressful as looking for something we're sure we saw an hour ago or the shame we feel about the state of a space. It can be overwhelming, though, so it's best done in tiny stages, bit by bit. Decluttering can apply to relationships; those that may be toxic, stressful or unhealthy.

12 DO THE BARE MINIMUM

It's all very much about the bare minimum right now. If you don't have any energy to wash, don't pile on the pressure about it – grab some wet wipes and some dry shampoo and make do with those for now. The same applies to all the things we feel we 'ought' to be doing – find the 'hack' – the lowest-energy way to address it. We can do better when we feel better.

When we feel low, we tend to give ourselves a hard time. There's a tendency to want approval from others; after all, we hardly approve of ourselves right now. What tends to happen then, though, is that we never jump out of the hamster wheel of life that has got us feeling so awful. It really is time to stop, to reflect and to streamline. The world really will wait if we ask it to. There's nothing as valuable, as precious or as important as our health – it can't be bought with more time or more money. Don't ignore the warning signs that life isn't working as it should. Take heed and make time to recover. We'll come back stronger for it.

Self-care for when we're scared, anxious and worried

There's nothing pleasant about feeling scared, anxious or worried, nothing at all. It's disruptive, exhausting, humiliating and debilitating. It can come out of nowhere, knock us to the floor and interrupt the best laid plans.

We've all experienced feeling this way and its knackering effects; the nervousness we feel before an exam or job interview, the tightness of our chests as we struggle to breathe, the flutter of nerves as we walk into a room full of people, the rush of panic when we have to speak in front of a group of people and the jitter we feel when we're worried about something.

For some of us, anxiety really plays havoc on our lives; it prevents us from socialising, from travel, from going to the dentist, from leaving the house.

There are a few things we can do as preventative measures, but also when we're in the throes of these feelings.

1 LISTEN TO MUSIC
Music is incredibly powerful; it's been shown to be able to increase, or decrease, our stress levels and heart rate. Our tastes in music are unique, only we know what soothes us, uplifts

or plays into our anger. By putting together a playlist of songs which soothe us, we can be prepared for when we get overturned by these worrisome feelings. If we have headphones, they can also work as a way of 'detaching' us from the external world just for a few moments until everything seems to have slowed down.

2 GO GENTLE

When we feel out of sorts, we tend to lay the blame at our door. We beat ourselves up and wish we were different. It gets us nowhere. If anything, it gives those thoughts legs, and we definitely don't want to do that. Whatever the reason we feel scared, worried or anxious, we wouldn't ever choose to feel that way. If we could only be a friend to ourselves in those moments, to pause and be as gentle as we would be to someone else who was struggling, the moment would pass quicker. Let's go gentle on ourselves and remember that we're doing our best.

3 HELP TO FORGE NEW PATTERNS

If we repeatedly find ourselves sidelined by these feelings and they're negatively impacting our lives, we might consider something called Cognitive Behavioural Therapy (CBT). CBT challenges our thoughts and teaches us new tools for coping with the situations which may cause us to be fearful and fretful. There are online platforms available: Living Life to the Full, MoodGym, Beating the Blues, Pacifica, or we can access it via a referral from our GP, or privately.

4 LIMIT CAFFEINE

Tea and coffee are embedded in our daily routines and we don't often pay them much thought, we enjoy drinking them and the pause in the day that having a cuppa incites. It's also a social activity for some. We know that drinking caffeine after 2 p.m. can affect our sleep quality but drinking caffeine full stop can exacerbate how we feel. The jittery feeling, that spike of energy, that we get from caffeine, can play right into the hands of those troublesome feelings of fear, worry and anxiety.

5 THERE'S AN APP FOR THAT

A shortness of breath increases the intensity of the fear, worry and anxiety we feel. It's frightening to find ourselves gasping for air and can be painful too. Many people feel as though they're experiencing a heart attack when they're in the middle of an anxiety attack.

For those of us who have experienced a shortness of breath in this way before, it's a good idea to install some apps on our smartphones which will guide us through these horrible spells. Some recommended apps are: Flowy, Mindshift, Breathe2Relax, Hear and Now.

6 DISTRACTION

When we feel the rumble of these feelings rise, it often acts as a catalyst for all the affirming worrisome thoughts and before we know it, we're overtaken by fear, stress and panic.

If we can distract ourselves early enough, we can dampen

these feelings before they dampen us. Again, as we tend to have our smartphones with us, there are some great apps to help with this: Flow Free, Panic Shield, What's Up?, Stress and Anxiety Companion.

But distractions can also be physical things we do to take our minds off the troubling thoughts. Some ideas include: knitting, colouring, solving puzzles, playing games, doodling, playing with a fidget spinner or sniffing some calming essential oils. These all take some prior planning to make sure we have them when needed.

Self-care for when we can't sleep

Sleep is crucial to how we function; it's when we mend, grow, process the day and get a much-needed break from everything.

The quality and quantity of our sleep can be affected by stress, health, life changes, what we may have eaten or drunk, medication, and our environment.

When sleep eludes us, we feel as though our warm and comfy bed havens are rejecting us – the bed suddenly feels so uncomfortable, our mind starts with all *those* thoughts again and the quiet loneliness of a 2 a.m. awake spell, when we're certain that everyone within our time-zone is getting some shuteye, makes each moment feel like an eternity.

We toss and turn to no avail. It's painful.

Let's look at some ways we can ease that frustration and aid our return to the Land of Nod.

1 MINIMISE LIGHT

Light, even a minimal amount, can play havoc with our quality of sleep. Our phones emit a blue light which suppresses the production of melatonin. Melatonin is the hormone which helps us to feel sleepy at the right time. When that's suppressed we may experience disrupted sleep. It's best to avoid our phones altogether when it's night-time and to look at how we can eradicate all electronic light too; the standby red light on the TV or stereo and alarm clock light. Consider wearing a sleep mask if you can't eradicate light altogether. We're programmed to sleep better in a dark, cool room.

2 BREATHE

Short shallow breathes are not conducive to sleep-mode. To lull ourselves back to sleep, we can forego counting sheep, and take note of the depth of our breath. The aim is to slow our breathing down by taking deeper, mindful breaths.

If that doesn't work, we can give visualisation a try. By visualising a beach, we can use the ebb and flow of the waves to steady our breathing. Watch as the wave recedes back and breathe in, in time with its journey back from the shoreline, then as it comes forward ready to break on the shore, we can slowly breathe out. Repeat until eyelids become heavy.

3 GET OUT OF BED

Clock-watching and calculating the hours until morning just wakes us up even more. We feel more panicked, more stressed and more awake. If it's been twenty minutes and we're still not sleepy, we might need to revisit some soothing activities until we feel tired again. That might be reading a book, listening

to some calming music or yoga – anything that promotes serenity
and makes us feel sleepy.

4 VENT

Those 2 a.m. thoughts are wily beasts, taking on a life of
their own in the early hours. It might be that the thoughts
are whirring about needlessly, and just need an output. It could
be that we've a solution to a problem whizzing about that just
needs to be captured. Whether it's ideas or worries that are
playing on our minds, offloading those thoughts into a notebook
can be incredibly freeing.

5 MAKE A WARM DRINK

Just as a warm shower or bath can relax us, the same can
be said for a mug of warm milk or chamomile tea. The act
of making the drink can be a distracting one and drinking it can
relieve the alertness we feel.

Reflect on the things you enjoyed as a child

_____

_____

_____

_____

_____

_____

_____

_____

_____

What's worrying you?
Brain-dump in the space below.

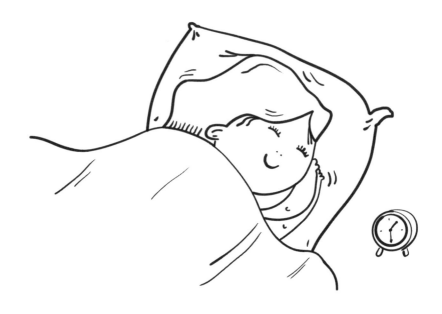

Consider your bedtime routine. How could it be tweaked to promote shuteye?

Self-care toolkit. What tools are in yours?

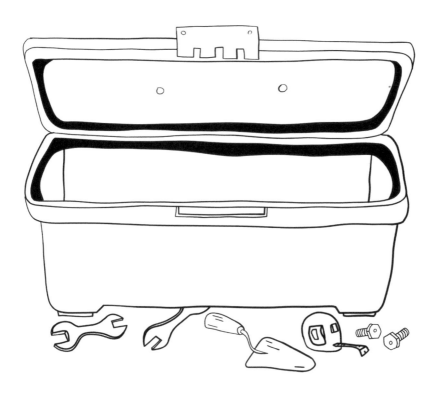

Your Emergency Self-Care Plan

○

○

○

○

○

○

○

○

○

A Letter from Me to You

Hey Twinkletoes,

You have just taken an almighty leap towards taking better care of yourself and that's no mean feat. Cue high fives, fist bumps, pats on the back, cartwheels and a big deep breath. I'm so proud of you because I know how difficult, uncertain and rickety that first step can be. You did it!

Whether your starting place was a good one or a grotty one, you're probably feeling a little overwhelmed by the changes you want to make, maybe a little surprised by some things you've unearthed about yourself and, hopefully, a little more understanding of your needs and how to elbow life out of the way to make room for those.

When the grotty times come, because they always do, know that you can and will get through them. Dig deep to find the diamonds of strength within you (I promise you that they're there), hold on tightly to those precious grains of hope and know that, one day, you'll look back at this and marvel at the courage, strength and determination you found within yourself. And know this, too: someone, somewhere, will be inspired by your act of bravery and will feel a glimmer of belief in themselves because of you.

Don't let the grotty times haunt you, either; they're gone for now.

Don't let them cast a shadow over who you are. Know that you have the tools to get through them when/if they return.

The rain will always ease off, the clouds will eventually float away, the dust will always settle.

Replace those sticks with which you beat yourself with soothing words of kindness. Look for the lessons within your mistakes. It's impossible that everything is your fault; other people exist and are learning, too. They'll make mistakes, you'll make mistakes, I'll make mistakes. You won't stop making mistakes, not if you're growing, but you can start to learn from them instead of collecting and carrying them on your shoulders.

Take good care of yourself – you're precious. You matter, you always have. You are incredible, exactly as you are right now.

Eke a little bit of yourself into your days and be prepared to blossom in ways that will astound you. It won't happen overnight but one day you'll look back and you'll see that you grew, you flourished, and that it only really took kindness to help you do it. The kindness from you to you.

Please fan the flame of your own being but don't burn out for others – show them how to fan their own flames. Be the example they need.

Continue the soothing and nurturing of your essence. The world needs what you, and only you alone, have to offer it. It's a much richer and more magical place because of you. Never doubt the difference you make, just by being you.

Your light shines so brightly. The thing about our luminosity is that it shines outwards like a lighthouse's beam does. You might not feel the benefits of your flame but rest assured we do. We see how brightly you shine. Just because you can't see it, doesn't mean it's not there, illuminating the lives of others, showering them in warmth and setting off a ripple of safety. Stand tall, wonderful one; you absolutely and unequivocally are enough. Exactly how you are right in this moment in time.

You deserve to twinkle, you deserve to shine. You deserve to be full to the brim with happiness. You deserve to be inspired, to feel effervescent. You deserve to live to see those dreams of yours come to fruition. You deserve all the world has to give, and more. You deserve it all.

And if you lose faith in yourself, you can borrow some of mine because my belief in you will never waver. I believe in you 100 squadillion per cent; I believe that you have exactly what it takes to get through anything and everything.

Sending a giant squishy hug.

Jayne x

These are a few of my favourite things

I try to curate what I see when I log into my personal social media feeds, so that it's inspiring and positive. It took me a long time to realise that I have control over what I see online and that social media is a tool that can both lift, but also make me feel pretty lousy. And that can change depending on how I'm feeling.

For those tough times, I've got some websites bookmarked which really have been lifesavers at times. For the better times, there are websites which help me explore who I am and help me on the path to how I'd like to be.

The aim is that rather than be a stick with which to beat myself, social media is more like a warm, cosy blanket.

I've put everything in a list for you, albeit a really varied list, in the hope it helps you to discover some gems too. Rather than list all their social media platforms too, you can click on the social media icons on their respective homepages to find those.

www.blurtitout.org

I was always going to have this website bookmarked, wasn't I?! I am truly proud of the content we produce and I find it really useful when I feel depression creeping towards me. It also helps to remind me that I'm not the worthless good-for-nothing that depression would have me believe I am.

Headspace: www.headspace.com
I find their blog articles incredibly insightful and they aid reflection.

Living Life: www.llttf.com
I've used the CBT modules many a time, and will continue to do so.

Samaritans: www.samaritans.org
I'm not ashamed to admit that I have called the Samaritans before and wouldn't hesitate to do so again – for a dose of empathy and advice in the darkest of times. Lifesavers.

I'm Alive: www.imalive.org
7 Cups of Tea: www.7cups.com
For the times anxiety has made using the telephone a really scary thing to do, I've used these sources of online support and they've been incredible. Lifesavers.

Self-Compassion: www.self-compassion.org
I am getting much better at practising self-compassion and find that reading this website helps me strive to be better at it. Always a work in progress, right?!

Thrive Global: www.thriveglobal.com
Don't we all want to thrive? I dip in and out of this website a lot as I love learning and reading other people's perspectives on some of the problems I face.

Quiet Revolution: www.quietrev.com
It took me years to realise that one of the reasons I didn't feel as though I fitted in was because I was an introvert with lots of extroverted friends. It's been liberating to learn about introversion and how schools, etc are biased towards extroversion.

Calm: www.calm.com
My go-to meditation and mindfulness app. I love that the recordings address the difficulties that we may have when we begin meditating – I don't find it easy at all and Tamara totally lets me off the hook for that which means I embrace the quiet and solitude with very little beating myself up going on.

The Mighty: www.themighty.com
My experiences of mental ill health have been predominantly depression and anxiety. The Mighty is an awesome platform where people share their experiences of mental ill health. I find the courage people show, inspiring. I also think we can learn a lot by listening to people and hearing about their experiences.

These are my favourite illustrators who are full of empathy and courage. They have a creative prowess that I hunker after. I mean, I once drew a robin and Peggy thought it was a kangaroo! I'm in awe of these creative geniuses and they make my social media feeds a better place to be.

Stacie Swift: www.stacieswift.com
Ruby etc: rubyetc.tumblr.com
Dallas Clayton: www.dallasclayton.com
Gemma Correll: www.gemmacorrell.com
Katie Abey: www. katieabey.co.uk
May The Thoughts be With You: www.maythethoughtsbewithyou.com
Sweatpants and Coffee: www.sweatpantsandcoffee.com
Mari Andrew: www.bymariandrew.com
Sonaksha Iyengar: sonaksha.tumblr.com

Being a Mum, a working Mum at that, is such a kaleidoscope of emotions. These fabulous ladies help me to feel less alone as they honestly and brilliantly talk about motherhood, with no holds barred. It's refreshing, and it's comforting, and I love it.

The Unmumsy Mum: www.theunmumsymum.co.uk
Mother Pukka: www.motherpukka.co.uk
Giovanna's World: www.giovannasworld.com
My Milo & Me: www.mymiloandme.com

Acknowledgements

There have been times when I have been so isolated and
misunderstood, that I've wanted to disappear. Times when I've
been so battered by depression that I've been empty, the smile
never reaching my eyes. Depression did a good job of convincing
me that the world would be better off without me, that it wouldn't
even miss me. I didn't dare dream that I would feel part of
something again, that I'd have friends, that I'd feel so loved.
To have the opportunity to sing loudly and proudly about
the people I am grateful for is one I'm going to embrace
wholeheartedly.

To Domski, words don't touch the sides when it comes to
expressing the gratitude I feel for you, words don't do justice
to the depth of love I have for you and the magnitude of how it
feels to be on the receiving end of your unwavering love for me.
Life hasn't always dealt you a fair hand – it's battered you and it's
bruised you – yet your love knows no bounds. There's a look you
have, I'm pretty sure that it's reserved just for me, and it says,
'I believe in you, I love you and I'll help you.' And you do. That look
of yours gives me strength. You believe in me when my self-belief
is running low. You love me when I'm at my most unlovable.
And you help me in so many ways: the hugs, the tear mopping,
the pom-pom shaking, the little notes you leave in my laptop,

the teamwork through the toughest times we've faced, the feeling that your life and mine were always meant to be entwined, the hand-holding as we navigate together the new paths we take through life. It's been a monumental privilege for me to walk through life at your side; there's nowhere I'd rather be. Thank you for choosing me. Thank you for letting me in. Thank you for trusting me with your heart – I promise it's in safe hands.

To Peggy, thank you for anchoring me. Being your mum is the most exquisite experience. You teach me so much more than I'll ever be able to teach you: the magic in the simple things, the power of an all-encompassing hug, that depression was lying to me when it said I'd be a terrible mum, that pride can lift me through the tougher times, that it's okay to stumble and crumble, the names of all the dinosaurs, and how to play again. You add so much sparkle to my days; I don't have the words to express just how much you mean to me, so I'm not even going to try. I hope you can feel it in your heart.

Next up is you, Mother Hubbs. How utterly blessed I am to have you as my mum. If I had to choose a mum, it would always be you. You astound me, and I hope I can be a smidgen of the mother to Peggy that you have been to me. You rocked motherhood and made it look so easy, even though I now know that it's often far from easy. Somehow, and I can't figure out how, you've simultaneously given me space to figure out who I am as well as surrounding me with safety. I've made some biiiig mistakes, but you're always so unflustered by them.
Your grace, patience and love have carried me on a gentle bobbing wave through some almighty storms. Thank you for all you are, all you've done and all you continue to be. You're my

biggest inspiration, and I'm so thankful too that you coaxed the writing back out of me. I'm not sure whose dream this book has fulfilled most – yours or mine. Perhaps my dreams are your dreams, just as Peggy's will one day be mine. When I grow up, I want to be just like you.

Motherhood has brought us closer together, Clairie Wairie Airy Fairy, and I am so happy that it has. I missed you during that weird time I think all siblings experience; the time of early adulthood when we grow wings and need to find our own feet. Hindsight has shown me how necessary that time was for you and me. I am so grateful that as fully fledged adults we grew back together. You no longer need a big sister to look out for you and my new role, as your friend, is one I cherish even more. Growing up with you has been so much fun. You taught me the power of perspective – that two people can experience the same thing but that their experience of that same thing can be different. I'm so glad that we still share a sense of humour that makes no sense to anyone else. One look from you is all it takes for the bubbles of giggles to rise, and usually at the most unfortunate of times. Your heart is so big, I have no idea how it fits inside your chest, and your loyalty knows no bounds. You've got my back, and I've got yours. Always.

Dadski, we've had a rocky ride of it, haven't we?! Love can be unconditional yet confusing. Love can be complicated, and it can't always be felt. It can hurt, and it can heal. I want you to know that you're lovelier than you know. I hope you'll one day loosen those fortress boundaries of yours to let more love in; you deserve to feel the love that is there for you. You did your best with what you knew; I know that now. You had wounds that wouldn't heal;

I know that now too. You're loved, much more than you realise, by us all.

Growing up with such a large family was magical, and I was never short of people to learn from and play with. They say that friends are the family we choose for ourselves but I've been lucky enough to have a family full of people who I would always have chosen as my friends. They're extraordinary. I want to say an extra-special thank you to Ammy, Keithie, Wendypops and Adgie. You know why.

To Stacie, Lotte, Maddy, Carlyn, Naomi, Steph, Jessy, Troy, Emma, Holly and Jo, a ginormous heartfelt thank you to each of you. It's an absolute honour to work with and become friends with you all. I pinch myself every day that work can be so fun and full of purpose. You're big-hearted, kind, generous, passionate and inspiring. I treasure you all. This book wouldn't even be a 'thing' without you – you've been magnificent brainstormers, sounding boards and fort-holders, and have championed its progress. Thank you so very much.

Abbie, you are a gigantic ray of sunshine. You came into my life and challenged everything that I thought was possible. Thank you for seeing something in me that I couldn't quite see at the time. Thank you for nurturing me, guiding me and teaching me. Thank you for your gentleness, patience and kickass pep talks. You've picked me up more times than you probably realise. Thank you for everything.

A giant thanks to Olivia and everybody at Orion Spring. Thank you for giving me a chance to put my ponderings about self-care into words, for holding my hand through the process, and for your astonishing commitment to this book. You're a gift

I dared not dream of having and I've learned so much from you. You made the experience of writing a book a fun, rewarding and exciting one. Thank you for believing in me.

At Blurt, we have a #nicestuff Slack channel, where we pop all the words of kindness and encouragement that we receive from the Blurt Fam. The #nicestuff comes at us from all angles; from social media, letters and cards we receive in the post, and emails. Each day, something new is added to the channel, and I can't express how powerful that has been; in helping me, and the amazing Blurt team, through uncertain times, dark times and times where I don't feel *I'm* doing enough. Thank you to everyone who has contributed to that channel – you have no idea how much you have lifted me, how powerful your voices have been against my harmful thoughts, and how much of a difference you have made. I'll keep working hard to make sure you're heard and understood.

blurt

BLURT EXISTS TO MAKE A DIFFERENCE TO ANYONE AFFECTED BY DEPRESSION

Being diagnosed can be overwhelming – there's a lot to learn and plenty of prejudice to battle. Telling people is tough, and not everyone will understand. That's why we're here for you, whenever you need us, for anything at all.

We'll help you to understand depression and what it means for you. We'll support you, listen to you and introduce you to people who've been where you are. We'll help you break down barriers and broach the subject with those closest to you. We'll help you help yourself, with a little knowing nod.

Find us online:

www.blurtitout.org
blurtitout
@blurtalerts
theblurtfoundation
blurtalerts

Share your self-care shenanigans,
self-care challenges, and 'a-ha!'
moments by using

#selfcareproject

across social media.